Praise for *The Success Trap*

"Achievement pressure is stressing young people out at epidemic levels. Dr. Stuart Slavin provides us here with a compelling, highly readable mix of research evidence, case stories, and potential solutions. I recommend the book to all parents, educators, and anyone else concerned with the mental wellbeing of young people."

—Peter Gray,
expert in childhood learning and author of *Free to Learn*

"*The Success Trap* is rigorous, urgent, and deeply practical, the road map every parent, educator, and school leader has been waiting for."

—Vicki Abeles,
New York Times bestselling author of *Beyond Measure*

"Stuart Slavin has done something rare and necessary: He has given us the science and the story behind a crisis hiding in plain sight. As both a pediatrician and a father, Slavin brings profound insight into how our culture's obsession with achievement is stealing childhood, adolescence, and even young adulthood away from us and harming the developing brain—creating unnecessary toxic stress and mental suffering. This book is a call to action for very parent, educator, and policymaker. Read it, share it, and let it change the way we support our youth on the challenging journey of staying grounded, connected, and inspired in their lives."

—Daniel J. Siegel,
New York Times bestselling author of
Brainstorm, Mind, and *Mindsight*

"A powerful explanation beyond 'It's the phones!' for why so many kids and teens seem to succeed in school but struggle in life. *The Success Trap* offers a blueprint—effective, economical, and actionable—for student success and well-being."

—Ned Johnson,
coauthor of *The Self-Driven Child*
and host of *The Self-Driven Child* podcast

"*The Success Trap* is a refreshing, necessary look at the reality of raising a child in today's success-driven, pressure-cooker society. Realistic, compassionate, and highly actionable, this book has the answers you've been looking for."

—**Julie Lythcott-Haims,**
New York Times bestselling author of *How to Raise an Adult*

"Dr. Slavin provides both a compelling account of the causes of distress among today's youth and practical pathways for fostering their well-being. Backed by solid research, he illuminates the pressures of our achievement-focused culture and offers realistic, evidence-based solutions. This is an essential guide for parents and educators who want to create environments in which young people can truly learn, thrive, and find meaning."

—**William R. Stixrud,**
coauthor of *The Self-Driven Child*
and founder of The Stixrud Group

"Many of us are looking for a new roadmap to success, aware that the old one is not just outdated but often harmful to teens. Dr. Slavin offers a compelling and comprehensive diagnosis of what's gone wrong and a path to turn things around. A practical and timely compass to help our teens navigate uncertain times."

—**Jenny Anderson,**
coauthor of *The Disengaged Teen*
and senior fellow for the Center for Teen Flourishing

"Stuart Slavin brings a powerful mix of clinical expertise and humane wisdom to bear on one of the deepest problems of our time. *The Success Trap* is a remarkable combination of social criticism and self-help—at once profound and useful."

—**Daniel Markovits,**
author of *The Meritocracy Trap*

THE SUCCESS TRAP

HOW THE PRESSURE TO STAND OUT IS FUELING ANXIETY, DEPRESSION, AND BURNOUT IN TEENS—AND THE FUNDAMENTAL FIX THEY DESERVE

STUART SLAVIN, MD, MEd

TEN SPEED PRESS
California | New York

Ten Speed Press
An imprint of the Crown Publishing Group
A division of Penguin Random House LLC
1745 Broadway
New York, NY 10019
tenspeed.com
penguinrandomhouse.com

Typefaces: Adobe's Garamond Pro and Monotype's Modica

Library of Congress Cataloging-in-Publication Data
Names: Slavin, Stuart J. author Title: The success trap: how the pressure to stand out is fueling anxiety, depression, and burnout in teens—and the fundamental fix they deserve / Stuart Slavin.
Identifiers: LCCN 2026005737 (print) | LCCN 2026005738 (ebook) | ISBN 9780593839386 hardcover | ISBN 9780593839416 trade paperback | ISBN 9780593839409 ebook Subjects: LCSH: Success in adolescence | Anxiety in adolescence | Teenagers—Mental health
Classification: LCC BF724.3.S9 S55 2026 (print) | LCC BF724.3.S9 (ebook)
LC record available at https://lccn.loc.gov/2026005737
LC ebook record available at https://lccn.loc.gov/2026005738

Hardcover ISBN 978-0-593-83938-6
Ebook ISBN 978-0-593-83940-9

Editor: Thea Diklich-Newell | Production editor: Ashley Pierce
Designer: Amani Shakrah | Production: Jessica Heim
Copy editor: Elizabeth Magnus | Proofreaders: Sigi Nacson and Miriam Taveras
Indexer: Ken DellaPenta | Publicist: Kristin Casemore | Marketer: Emily Hotaling

Manufactured in the United States of America

1st Printing

First Edition

To my parents, Raymond and Alberta Slavin,
who instilled in me a desire to do some good in the world.

This book contains references to suicide and mental health struggles, which may be distressing to some readers.

If you or someone you know is struggling or in crisis, help is available: Call or text 988 to reach the Suicide and Crisis Lifeline for free, confidential support 24/7.

The information in this book is provided for educational purposes and is not a substitute for medical or mental health advice, diagnosis, or treatment. If you have concerns about your child's mental health, please seek guidance from a qualified mental health or other health care professional.

Contents

Introduction *xi*

Part 1
Achievement Culture Is Harming Our Kids

Chapter 1
The Adolescent Mental Health Crisis: It's Not Just About Tech *3*

Chapter 2
Depression in the Age of Pressure: What Every Parent Should Know *27*

Chapter 3
Understanding Anxiety: When Normal Worry Turns to Distress *46*

Part 2
A Case Study

Chapter 4
My Initiative to Combat Depression, Anxiety, and Toxic Stress in My Students *71*

Part 3
Finding Solutions

Chapter 5
Problematic Mindsets: The Thought Patterns That Can Trap Kids *95*

Chapter 6
Cognitive Distortions: How Unhelpful Thoughts Can Amplify Distress *123*

Chapter 7
Goal Disruption Theory: Why Many Kids Crash Out When Things Don't Go Their Way *149*

Chapter 8
Your Kid in School: Too Much, Too Fast—And Why Kids Feel Disengaged *166*

Chapter 9
Your Kid After School: The Overcommitment Trap *194*

Chapter 10
Giving Kids More Control, More Choice, and Opportunities to Find Connection, Meaning, and Joy *219*

Conclusion *247*
Supplemental Resources *251*
Acknowledgments *268*
Notes *272*
Index *285*

Introduction

It was 7:30 in the evening, and the golden light of a warm spring day was beginning to fade as I picked up my daughter from her tennis team practice. She was nearing the end of her junior year in a private high school in St. Louis, Missouri. She clambered into the car, slumped back in her seat, and let her shoulders drop. I didn't need to be a physician to see that she was completely exhausted, so I held in my cheerful questions about her day and we made the five-minute drive home in silence. We could catch up later. But as we walked in the front door, she ran straight up the stairs toward her room, leaving me watching her retreating figure. "Dinner's ready!" her mom called out, and we heard her yell back, "I don't have time, I have so much homework to do." When my wife and I pressed her to join us, our daughter broke into tears and said, "You don't understand—I literally don't have time to eat!"

This incident wasn't a one-off event or in any way unusual. My daughter had been working at a breakneck speed with school, extracurricular activities, and homework since the beginning of ninth grade, regularly putting in sixteen-hour days that barely let up on weekends or holidays. Originally, we had been drawn to her school by its reputation as St. Louis's most progressive school, where values of social justice, equity, and inclusion were embraced and all the students called the faculty and staff by their first names. It was a place that seemed to appreciate and encourage curiosity and creativity. We were completely charmed when we first walked through the front door for a student recruitment evening: Artwork covered the high walls of the large entryway; the school jazz band was riffing away; and a racially diverse group of parents gathered around, chatting—not a typical sight in what remained a largely segregated city. The first two years in junior high were lovely for our family. Our daughter found great friends, we met like-minded parents, and the teachers were bright and engaging. She was happy, and so were we. While busy with her schoolwork, she had time to spend with her family and friends.

Things changed abruptly with the start of ninth grade. The pace of the school day, the amount of homework, and the expectations and achievement pressures all ramped up as the administration and teachers made it clear to the students that their grades would now be on their "permanent record" for the college application process. It wasn't just the change in grade level, the move from junior high to high school, that contributed to the increase in demands. There was a sea change in the academic requirements, a concerted effort to intensify the curriculum to make it more rigorous, a change designed in part to attract more affluent families with their sights set on prestigious colleges. The entranceway, while still displaying a wonderful array of student artwork, now featured a large poster that read, "WHERE WILL YOUR SAT SCORE TAKE YOU?"

I observed my daughter's experience in the ninth and tenth grades, not just as a concerned parent, but also as a pediatrician and medical educator. I could see that what was being asked, or *demanded,* of her and her peers—a nightly homework load of three hours or more plus extracurricular sports, clubs, and endless rehearsals for the school play—seemed completely unreasonable and developmentally inappropriate for fourteen- to sixteen-year-old kids. It wasn't all bad—the visual arts program was superb, the athletics programs were fairly low-key, the head of school was a thoughtful and principled person, and the teachers were by and large a dedicated and talented group—but these positives did not negate the reality that the demands and pressure were too great.

Expectations escalated even more in the eleventh grade. The jam-packed seven periods per day continued from her earlier years but were now accompanied by an even greater amount of homework, brought on by the four Advanced Placement (AP) courses she was taking—a perceived minimum if she wanted to be considered by an elite college. Relaxing weekends and a full night's sleep were a thing of the past. On top of her academic load were sports practices, games, and meets during two of the three sports seasons, rehearsals and performances for school drama productions, membership in and leadership of clubs and interest groups, community service, and the beginning of the college search and application process, including SAT practice and tests. My daughter was, and is, tough, smart, driven, and resilient, but at times school, and all that came with it, was just too much. She would go to bed late, only to get up early the next morning to do it all over again. It was relentless, and there was a visible toll on her as well as on our family. She often had bouts of impatience, short-temperedness, and even, on occasion, meltdowns—and who could blame her? She was completely burned out. My wife and I and her younger sister often felt like we were walking on eggshells, trying to avoid conflict or burdening her with anything extra. There is a saying that a parent is only as happy as their least happy child, and that was certainly the case for us.

What made it even more difficult was that my wife and I felt helpless to protect her from all this. As a pediatrician, I knew the importance of getting adequate sleep and the negative long-term effect that her late nights coupled with early mornings would have on her mental, physical, and cognitive health. I had read the concerning medical literature on depression, anxiety, and suicide in teens and young adults and knew that the outrageous expectations placed on her—and her classmates—were likely harmful.

As a concerned parent and board member at the school, I made repeated entreaties over several years to the head of school and the board to decrease academic demands and reduce the pressure, as our kids were staggering under the weight of a curriculum that was needlessly and senselessly burdensome. I was a big believer in a challenging education, critical thinking, and healthy competition, and I wanted my daughter to feel driven to do her best in her academic and extracurricular pursuits—just not at the expense of her well-being. Unfortunately, my arguments for academic rigor without the relentless pressure didn't land, even when they came from the angle of a pediatrician concerned for the well-being of all the kids, not just my own daughter's. I was politely listened to but action didn't follow. The prevailing notion was that the hours of daily homework were necessary to make the students competitive in the high-stakes race to college. It was the only way to set them up for success.

I came to realize that I would not be able to effect change at my daughter's school, a dispiriting feeling that I believe many parents in this country have experienced. The reality is that it's hard to transform an environment alone when we're dealing with entrenched societal attitudes about work, productivity, and the definition of success—what it means to achieve the American Dream. In the end, I stopped my entreaties and we stayed at the school, making it through another grueling year to graduation, before sending our daughter off to college. But my concerns didn't go away. I vowed that I would not give up fighting for change at other schools, in other communities. I knew in my gut that the excessive demands we were placing on our kids were wrong.

During the time that I watched my daughter suffer at school, I was working with another highly stressed group of students as the associate dean for curriculum at Saint Louis University (SLU) School of Medicine. By conducting surveys there, we had found that the heavy workload and high expectations placed on our medical students by the school were seriously affecting their mental health, contributing to high rates of depression and anxiety. My response at SLU (pronounced slew) was to figure out solutions to alleviate depression and anxiety in our students while still maintaining rigorous academic standards—which resulted in one of the most effective preventive mental health interventions ever documented

(I'll share details later in the chapter and throughout the book). It wasn't too much of a stretch to apply the same findings to a younger demographic of high schoolers. My successful experience at SLU, which followed hard on the heels of my daughter's high school years, inspired me to turn my attention to teen mental health—to explore the research, conduct my own studies, find answers, and, ultimately, write this book.

Changes are desperately needed, as the reality is that we are in the midst of a youth mental health emergency, one that former surgeon general Vivek Murthy described as the "defining public health crisis of our time." Multiple studies have documented rising rates of depression and anxiety in teens. In 2023, the National Survey on Drug Use and Health (NSDUH) found that 18.1 percent of adolescents aged twelve to seventeen had had a major depressive episode in the past year,[1] and the National Survey of Children's Health showed that 16.1 percent of adolescents ages twelve to seventeen had a current diagnosis of an anxiety disorder.[2]

I have targeted this problem in my own research, conducting, over the past decade, surveys of more than eighteen thousand teenagers in eighteen high schools (and one university) in three different states to explore depression, anxiety, daily life, and teens' ratings of different stressors in their lives. I wanted to go directly to the young people themselves to understand how they are handling unprecedented academic pressure and the relentlessly high expectations placed on them. In my studies, I have consistently found far higher rates of mental illness compared to the national data. Since 2013, in conjunction with my work in medical education and well-being, I've had the opportunity to travel the country and speak with a multitude of people—young and old—about youth mental health. While my primary professional focus was on medical students, medical residents, and faculty, I was able to dedicate time to also explore adolescent mental health. I've listened to parents, teachers, principals, superintendents, board members, coaches, pediatricians, psychologists, social workers, school nurses, psychiatrists, and mental health experts—people who work with and care about children and teens—and, most importantly, to teens themselves.

This is what I've found in my surveys *and* my conversations: A key contributor to the teen mental health crisis in many communities in this country is the pressure-cooker conditions that we have created for our kids. They are struggling under the crushing weight of school and extracurricular demands, of performance and achievement pressure placed on them by teachers, coaches, parents, themselves, and our society itself—and it's only getting worse. The overpressurized and stressful school and extracurricular environment that my daughter experienced some years ago has spread. I believe that a phenomenon that two decades ago was largely concentrated in private and public high schools in affluent urban and suburban communities, particularly in large cities on the East and West Coasts, and documented extensively by researcher Suniya Luthar[3] and author and psychologist Madeline Levine,[4] has proliferated, expanding in a slow-motion contagion into every state, infecting a wider and wider socioeconomic swath, and moving ever earlier within the K-12 continuum.

In large part, this spread is driven by parental fear in the face of economic uncertainty in a quickly changing world. Parents are under enormous pressure to provide what is best for their kids, to launch them on a path to success—defined by financial stability, material possessions, and social status. As income and wealth disparities have grown in recent years and as the middle class has shrunk, for many families the promise of this rosy future seems less and less likely. Many parents today realize that their kids are at risk of being less well off than they are, and they feel they must therefore do all they can to ensure that their child has the best chance possible of landing among the "haves" rather than the "have-nots."

Ultimately, this means a scramble for places in top colleges, still viewed as a reliable launching pad into the top echelons of future success—and so begins the race for kids to stand out from their peers, to rack up accomplishments, accolades, and achievements to catch the eye of admissions directors, to gather what writer David Brooks refers to as "résumé virtues."[5] The fear and social pressure that parents face are powerful, and they lead many parents to make choices about schools and promote after-school activities that are ostensibly for the good of their kids but that only add to the pressures and demands that they already face. I have spoken with many parents who have confided that they don't feel comfortable with the harried, stressful lives they've encouraged their kids to lead, that they feel trapped in cages of their own making, but that there doesn't seem to be an alternative or a way out. I know exactly how they feel.

As a researcher and physician who has spent my career interacting with children, teens, and young adults, I can't help but wonder if we've moved the goalposts of success too far, asking more and more of our kids, and, in doing so, have lost sight of what a "successful" childhood looks like. When did we decide that acceptance at a selective college should be our all-encompassing goal or allow college admissions directors to dictate how our teens spend their time and energy? When did we collectively agree to strive for eighteen years in the relentless pursuit of so-called success? The pressure of achievement culture comes with great potential risks for kids, including anxiety, depression, and suicidality, and the loss of the simple joys and independence of childhood. We need to ask ourselves if we're willing to open ourselves up to these dangers when we pursue the dreams we have for our children. We need to consider whether the quest for success has become a trap.

In my hands-on experience at SLU, my research, and my travels, I have developed a deep knowledge of the nature of the toxicity of the educational and social environments that many of our kids live in, the academic and extracurricular demands that, together, create an unhealthy achievement culture. Parents have told me stories of this world—an eighth grader who was devastated, crying for hours in his bedroom, because of an A minus on a quiz, a seventh-grade girl who refuses to go to school because of the unbearable pressure to be perfect that she feels there, and two bright teenage brothers who have essentially opted out of the system and are now getting a mix of Ds and Fs on their report cards. From the time they were babies, many of our kids have absorbed the message of achievement culture; that they must aim for the top, strive for perfection, do more, and do it better, that only then will they be successful or happy, and that anything less is abject failure. They are on a hamster wheel chasing grades and prizes, and it's making them sick.

In *The Success Trap,* I'll share my insights with you so that you too can understand the problem and begin to implement solutions. The stories and descriptions will be familiar to many of you, and the answers I propose—the steps we can all take—are simple to grasp and apply and may make the critical difference in stemming this youth mental health crisis that continues to surge.

Digital technology and social media have been in many ways singled out as *the* culprits for the decline in teen mental health, but when I talk to parents, that doesn't completely ring true to them. Yes, many are concerned and think their kids could benefit from less time on their screens and more time experiencing real life, but they view the outrageous academic and extracurricular demands and pressure their kids face as equally harmful. And they feel trapped, caught in a web of societal norms of overachievement and scared that if they opt out or step back their kids' futures will be compromised, that they'll miss out on their chance of attaining the American Dream. Many, if not all, are searching for solutions to a problem they feel helpless to solve.

In the chapters that follow, I'll explore three broad domains that, according to research (including my own), collectively contribute to much of the distress and struggle that many teens (and younger children) are experiencing:

1. Excessive school and extracurricular demands and pressure
2. Problematic mindsets and distorted thought patterns
3. A lack of joy, meaning, choice, and control in teenagers' lives

The good news is that in each of these areas change and progress are possible and collectively can have a huge positive impact on kids' and parents' lives.

Excessive Demands and Pressure

I'll explore how a rise in demands on our kids' energy and time has been accompanied by an unprecedented increase in pressure to achieve and to stand out from the competition—often in service of a mistaken idea that parents must launch their child to the most prestigious college possible or their future success will be forever compromised.

I'll show that the pressures that our kids are facing at earlier and earlier ages in school and in extracurricular activities are excessive and harmful—contributing to anxiety, depression, suicidal ideation, insomnia, and disordered eating. The increases in demands have been driven by the incorrect notion that adding more of some factor will always lead to better outcomes—for example, if one hour of homework is good, imagine our kids' performance if they had three or more hours! As I'll explain later in the book, there is no human endeavor in which more always leads to better outcomes—at some point, performance levels off and then begins to deteriorate, along with mental health.

However, as challenging as this situation may be—especially as the momentum appears to be going in the wrong direction—there is a solution, and it's as simple as it is potentially powerful. Reduce demands, reduce pressure, and not only is mental health likely to improve for a great many teens, but their academic performance is likely to get better as well. In the chapters that follow, I'll show you how this can work.

Problematic Mindsets and Distorted Thought Patterns

As many parents and educators share with me when I talk with them, a huge source of the pressure that kids feel comes *from within.* I've had parents tell me about their elementary school–aged children (as young as six!) falling apart because of a less-than-perfect score on a quiz or homework assignment, even though they have told their child that they don't care about their scores on these silly tests. Or high-achieving teens who panic before tests in case they ruin their perfect GPA. Many kids and teens suffer from problematic mindsets; these include maladaptive perfectionism and toxic comparison, as well as distorted thought patterns, such as magnification (taking a relatively small event and blowing it up into something huge) and all-or-nothing thinking. These mental models, stories, and self-narratives intersect with the demanding environments that kids live in and compound their distress, creating a vicious cycle of toxic stress.

I'll introduce the mindsets and thought patterns that are common in kids these days (and that you will likely recognize in yourself as well) and explain how you can help your kids manage them. The really good news is that not a single one of these mindsets and distorted thinking patterns is fixed—they can all be changed. I'll discuss ways to increase resilience and coping mechanisms in the face of stress, which, after all, is part of modern living.

Of course, children and teens don't come by their mindsets independently, and I'll explore two components that contribute to or initiate their maladaptive thinking: namely, parental mental models and societal conditioning. Parents have their own operative mindsets and internal narratives that feed their own questions and worries, which then affect their child's. *Am I doing enough to assure my child's path to success and happiness?* Or, to amplify this question, *Am I outdoing everyone else on that score? Do I have a soccer coach and a math tutor for my six-year-old? If not, maybe I'm not a good parent. Is my daughter enrolled in extracurricular STEM classes or summer camps? Would fencing or judo help my child stand out more on a college application?* For many parents, the pressure to be a model parent starts well before their child enters school. Indeed, it can begin immediately after the positive pregnancy test. In a competitive world, parents feel they need to optimize every moment of childhood to set their child on the path to success, from prestigious preschool to elite college. By the time the high school years come along, the pressure often reaches a fever pitch as preparations build toward the culmination of this master plan.

There are alternatives to this narrow, overly prescribed path, but choosing them takes courage. I'll offer possibilities and share ways that parents can push through their doubts and fears to try a different, more balanced approach, giving you the confidence to do less, and to say no to a system that asks too much.

Lack of Joy, Meaning, Choice, and Control

Many of the kids I have spoken with during my travels have painted a stark picture of the lack of meaning and joy in their lives. School and after-school activities have become work, an endless parade of days filled with relentless productivity and stress. And it isn't just what has been added that is a problem; it is what has been lost. The experience of childhood itself has been compromised. Kids often have little to no choice or control in their lives about what or how they are learning or how they are spending their time. Opportunities for in-person connection or downtime, just hanging out with peers, are severely limited. Time to pursue their own interests, to read a book or pursue a hobby for pleasure, has disappeared. Joy rarely appears, and when it does, it is often a fleeting experience at best.

The solutions are fairly simple—stop overcurating kids' experiences, free up time and space in their lives, and provide opportunities for them to find joy and meaning in compelling activities of their own choosing.

I wrote this book primarily for parents of teens and preteens (and for others who care for children); at its heart it's a parenting book. I also hope that it finds its way into the hands of some teens, who may see their experience captured in it. In my conversations with parents of even younger children from across the country, I have increasingly realized that pressure culture has trickled down to middle and elementary school years, and I believe parents with kids in this age group could also benefit. Finally, I hope that administrators, teachers, and coaches in K-12 education will take to heart the evidence and the recommendations offered here and enact much-needed and overdue changes that have the potential to improve the mental health of our youth.

Throughout the book my aim is to empower you to do what's really right for your child and for your family, to free yourselves from the traps you've unwittingly become ensnared in. In light of that, I'm especially excited to share a crucial outcome of my initiative at SLU, beyond the dramatic improvements in mental health and well-being. Though SLU students spent an hour and a half to two hours *less* each day in class or studying than the average U.S. medical student, their academic performance not only did not diminish; it actually *rose*! This fact disproved the widely held belief that greater demands and pressure produce better academic outcomes. If reducing workloads and pressure can lead to better mental health without compromising academic outcomes, who can argue against those changes?

I practiced pediatrics for twenty-one years at UCLA (including four years of training there), and one of the most important, and gratifying, things I did was provide anticipatory guidance to parents on how to raise a happy, healthy child. I offered them the information, based in science and my experience, that I thought they needed to make good decisions, and then the choice was theirs. Use time-outs, don't use time-outs? I would let parents know why they could be useful—time-outs allow a child to learn to self-regulate when they are falling apart—but ultimately the decision to use them or not was up to the parents.

In this book, I take a similar approach, describing the problems in our system and culture and their impact on our kids, bringing in the latest science and evidence, and providing specific, actionable, feasible interventions; but I leave it up to you, the parent, to determine which advice is most relevant to you as you guide your child along a happier, healthier path. My hope is that the stories I share, from my patients and my research, as well as from my own experiences and those of other parents and teens, will resonate with you, helping you see that you're not alone in feeling the stresses and concerns you do and that alternatives are available.

My aim is that by the end of the book you will feel supported and better armed—with information and practical strategies—to help your child navigate a path to success *and* good mental health. After all, it's hard to have the first without the second. I also hope that some of your own concerns and fears will lessen. In my pediatric practice, I found that many parents (especially new parents) experienced worry and uncertainty and, at times, an existential questioning of their parenting: *Am I a good parent? Am I doing it right?* When I affirmed parenting approaches or taught new ones, I could often see the worry on the faces of the parents melt away as they grew more comfortable with the choices they were making. I hope that, as you read, you will have a similar experience: that your doubts and apprehensions will be lessened, that you'll reassess where you stand, and that you'll begin to see how best to move forward in a way that prioritizes your child's mental health.

Many parents I have spoken with in recent years have voiced their intuitive sense that there was something wrong with the larger environment in which their child was struggling, whether to excel, keep up, or simply survive. So many of us have felt unsure about what's best for our child in a society that demands so much of them—and of us. Perhaps you are one of those parents, and you have longed for a road map to help guide your family forward in a way that feels balanced and advocates for your child's happiness in addition to their success. My overarching hope for *The Success Trap* is that it will show you such a path—or, perhaps, more accurately, offer you the tools, based on evidence (both scientific and anecdotal), to choose your own path, one that's best suited to your unique child.

As you'll see, there's much you can do as a parent, both within your home and outside of it, that can safeguard, or restore, a sense of wholeness to your child's life and yours. For those of you who aspire to do more—to lead the charge, or be part of the charge, that creates enduring change within your community's school and achievement culture, I provide a guide for this as well. I'm hopeful that you'll take the ideas in this book and use them to reintroduce joy and meaning to your kids, to bring about change that allows them to be excited and empowered by challenges rather than beaten down by pressures. Many of the stories in this book that were shared by parents, educators, and kids speak to this possibility. They also speak to the importance of integrating space and freedom into the lives of kids and families, unpacking previously too-full, too-stressful lives, and finding ways to redefine success. In ways big and small, they heed the warning of Socrates—"Beware the barrenness of a busy life"—and, in doing so, reimagine what childhood and adolescence can look like.

Part 1

Achievement Culture Is Harming Our Kids

Chapter 1

The Adolescent Mental Health Crisis: It's Not Just About Tech

There is little disagreement among researchers, mental health professionals, and policy makers that we have a teen mental health crisis on our hands; however, there is significant debate about the cause. In recent years, a number of prominent voices, including former U.S. surgeon general Vivek Murthy, social psychologist and author Jonathan Haidt, and psychologist and researcher Jean Twenge, have attributed the reason for this emergency to the rise in use of digital technology, especially social media, among children and adolescents, and in Haidt's case to a simultaneous decline in real-world opportunities for free play in childhood. They have a compelling theory, one that resonates with many of us, as examples of each abound in our lives; our kids' curated schedules combined with too much screen-based activity, and their many attendant ills, bear little resemblance to the childhoods that some of us remember so fondly. And yet, as appealing as it is to embrace one cause, or a pair of dovetailing causes, the story of how this increase in teen mental illness developed and took hold of a great swath of adolescents is, I believe, far more complex.

In this chapter, I'll review some of the evidence that links social media and digital technology use to an increase in teen distress and offer you an additional view based in my own research and others', one that will ring true for many of you: namely, that in many communities across the country and around the globe, it is school and extracurricular demands and achievement pressure that are driving this crisis. I'm not saying that social media and technology aren't a problem, far from it; I believe that they are, especially when combined with academic pressure. But if we focus only on a single cause, we miss being able to address something that has been hiding in plain sight for years—that we demand way too much of our kids in school and extracurricular activities, and it's taking a serious toll on them.

Jonathan Haidt's bestseller *The Anxious Generation: How the Great Rewiring of Childhood Is Causing an Epidemic of Mental Illness* has drawn tremendous attention to how rampant and pervasive digital technology use is among teens, and even children, and how detrimental it can be to their developing minds.[1] As he points out, it has unbalanced—to say the least—the foundations of childhood and family life. Wherever we look, it seems that we can find groups of kids and young adults, heads buried in their phones, their minds far away from the world around them. Educators struggle to compete with devices to maintain the attention of their students, and parents worry about kids who are lost to online content and exposed to porn, hate, and violence, yet have little understanding of how to pull them back or keep them safe. They sense that so much screen time and the corresponding loss of in-person connection is undermining their children in multiple ways but feel ill equipped to deal with the problem. I agree with much that Haidt has to say and welcome his and others' expertise on the subject. I believe that some aspects and impacts of screen-based activities and social media are problematic and are very likely contributing to the rise in mental illness in teens. I believe, however, that we are remiss when we fail to acknowledge that for some young folks social media provides a lifeline as they find "their people" in online groups. Many of Haidt's policy recommendations make good sense to me, such as banning smartphone use in schools, as does his parenting advice, including creating device-free times, waiting as long as possible before giving your teen a smartphone, and reclaiming family time. I agree with his assertion that free (meaning unsupervised by an adult) play has virtually disappeared from childhood and that this lack of time and space to explore, to practice being in relationship with others, and to enjoy being a kid is having profound negative downstream consequences—social, physical, and intellectual—that carry into adulthood.

However, I do not believe that the use of digital technology by kids, and the world it has been instrumental in shaping for them, is the *only* driver of our teen mental health crisis, or even the primary driver in some communities. Other important forces are also at play, and we neglect them at our peril. I'll begin by addressing what I see as the limitations of a position that only focuses on tech and obscures a deeper and more complex understanding of the threats to teens' mental health—why they often feel so stressed, unworthy, and ill equipped to carry on in their current lives, let alone transition into adult life.

Looking at the Evidence

A key element of Haidt's theory rests on a sharp increase in teen depression and anxiety rates starting in 2010 that coincides with a rise in smartphone use and what he refers to as a phone-based childhood. He asserts that the dramatic upsurge in the use of tech was the *only* major societal shift at the time that could have produced such a huge increase in mental illness, so, perforce, smartphones and the digital world *must* be the cause. While the evidence he brings forward may seem compelling, I have several concerns with this viewpoint.

Depression in Teens over the Decades

Haidt uses various graphs to illustrate his point, including one that tracks depression rates in girls and boys ages twelve to seventeen from 2004 to 2023. I took that same data, combined the boys and girls, and created the graph below.

The data is from the National Survey on Drug Use and Health (NSDUH), conducted by the Substance Abuse and Mental Health Services

Percentage of 12- to 17-Year-Olds with
Major Depressive Episode (MDE) by Year

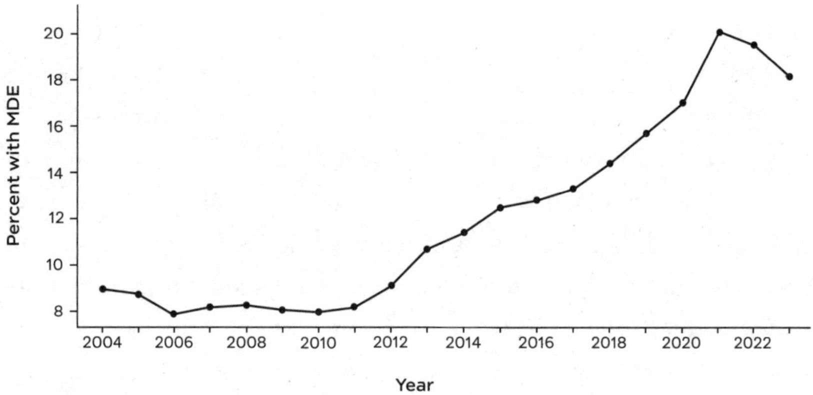

Administration (SAMHSA), and reports the percentage of that age group who have suffered at least one major depressive episode in the past year, which is a proxy for depression rate. Before delving into this data, it's important to state that this rise in depression is not a new trend, as the graph seems to suggest. Teen depression rates were *not* stable for a long stretch of time prior to a dramatic uptick in 2010. The graph starts in 2004, the year when the NSDUH survey began asking about depression, and Haidt used this dataset for good reason—it is rare to have such high-quality measurements of depression across a twenty-year span. That said, to have a full picture of teen depression and its cause(s), we need to have some idea of what was happening during the years *before* 2004, and for that we must turn to other data sources and research. While there are not the same high-quality measures stretching over the previous decades, there is strong evidence and general scientific consensus that the mental health of teens and young adults has been in steady decline for years—from long before the widespread adoption of smartphones—and this is supported by multiple studies. One such study, published in 2005, analyzed data from a national survey of outpatient (clinic) visits by kids aged seven to seventeen years.[2] They found that between 1995 and 2002, the number of visits for depression more than doubled, from 1.44 million to 3.22 million.[3]

Researcher Jean Twenge, who in recent years has become a strong proponent of the link between screens and poor mental health, was lead author on two studies that provide evidence that mental illness has been on the increase for decades. The first examined data from studies of teens from 1951 to 2002, utilizing the Minnesota Multiphasic Personality Inventory (MMPI), which includes questions about mental health.[4] Twenge found significant increases in scores on mental illness scales, including depression, and she concluded that adolescent mental illness rose considerably over that time period. A second study by Twenge looked at data from the Monitoring the Future survey from 1982 to 2012, in which nationally representative groups of twelfth graders in the U.S. were asked about physical symptoms that could accompany depression, including sleep issues, trouble with memory, difficulty thinking, and shortness of breath when not exercising.[5] A substantial increase in these symptoms was found across the entire thirty years of the study, and the rise was not limited to the last few years when smartphones made their appearance in teens' lives. Twenge attributed the mental health decline in young people to several factors—reduced autonomy (lacking the capacity to have choices in life), a rise in extrinsic motivation (being motivated by outside factors like grades and money) and a fall in intrinsic motivation (being motivated by a personal sense of meaning or purpose), a decline in free play that preceded digital technology, and an increasing cultural emphasis on money and status as symbols of success. These are all elements that I'll return to later in the book.

The evidence indicates that, despite a flat period between 2004 and 2010, depression and other mental illnesses in teens have seen a marked upward trend since the 1950s, not just since the introduction of smartphones and the rise of digital technology in daily life. In other words, the spike in the graph does not tell the whole story. Other factors have been harming teen mental health for decades—and it makes sense to continue to be open-minded to all possible causes.

Correlation Versus Causation

Much of the evidence used by researchers shows correlation but does not prove causation. Smartphone use and rates of teen mental illness have indeed both risen in sync during the same period, so one can say that they are temporally *correlated*—they happened at the same time. This is not in and of itself evidence of *causation,* of one being responsible for the other. Let me give you an example of two other things that have strong temporal correlations: ice cream consumption and drownings. They both show marked rises in the summer months and decreases in the winter months, and their parallel ups and downs could be plotted on a graph; however, no one would assert that eating ice cream causes drowning. I'm not suggesting that the smartphone/youth mental health crisis theory is wrong, just that it isn't conclusive and therefore that there is plenty of room for other causes of or contributors to our teens' diminishing mental well-being—so let's not close off other avenues of exploration.

What Else Might Contribute to the Rise in Mental Illness?

Haidt asserts that the dramatic rise in mental illness in young adults could only have been caused by the use of tech and social media (and a decline in free play). Others disagree. Some have pointed to climate change, ongoing global crises, or gun violence as major stressors that could have played a part. In a critical review of Haidt's book in the journal *Nature,* Candice Odgers, a well-respected developmental and quantitative psychologist, stated that the Great Recession of 2007 to 2009, and the unemployment and economic uncertainty that occurred in its aftermath, could have contributed to the mental health decline we have seen.[6]

Some have dismissed Odgers's theory because unemployment rates were coming down even as teen depression rates were rising, but I believe that she is on the right track. The recession and its reverberations are part of a larger economic picture in the U.S. of a widening gap in wealth and income between the upper classes and everyone else. This growing disparity has fueled a fear of being left behind on the part of parents and kids alike, who sense that the American Dream is growing further out of reach. This has led to enormous pressure to gain entry into an elite or at least a highly selective college, since such schools are still considered a gateway to financial and social success. I believe that the intense educational demands and relentless pressures seen as necessary to achieve that goal are fueling a rise in rates of mental illness and have been for some time. Once largely limited to elite high schools in wealthy communities, achievement pressure has spread, a contagion of competition, to affect a wider socioeconomic swath across the country. In turn, the perceived paths to success have narrowed and decreased in number, and the race to qualify in order to even compete begins earlier and earlier in the timeline of childhood.

How Depression Tracks with Pressures to Compete

To illustrate my point, I'd like to present several graphs that show societal trends alongside the depression rates in adolescents from the graph that I shared with you before. You may be surprised by what they reveal.

First let's plot depression (the solid line) along with the average number of college applications made per student on the Common App platform since 2014, when data first became available (the dashed line).[7] Applications began to rise as competition for places heated up—and you'll see that depression rates rose too, keeping pace.

Teen Depression vs. Avg. College Applications per Student (2014–2023)

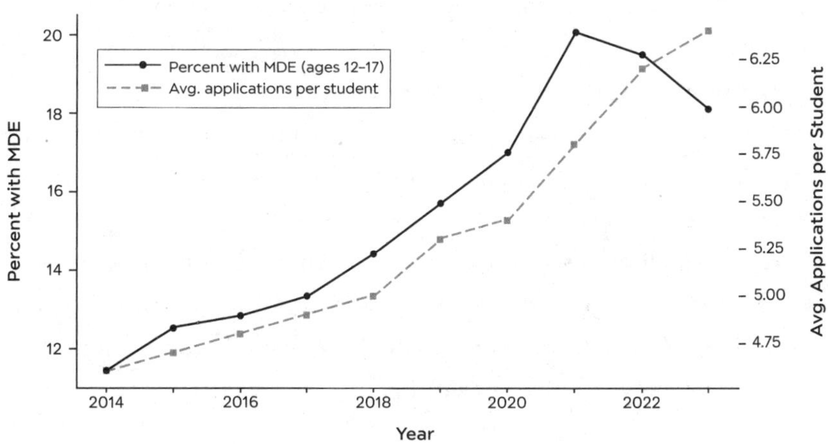

It isn't just the average number of applications that has increased, the percentage of students applying to more than ten schools has risen dramatically as well, more than doubling from 8 percent in 2014–15 to 17 percent in 2021–2022.

As the number of applications has increased, the pursuit of metrics to bolster applications has intensified. Students are keen to prove their academic prowess and stand out from the crowd, often by taking Advanced Placement (AP) courses and exams. Here is depression (the solid line) graphed with the number of AP tests taken annually (the dashed line).[8]

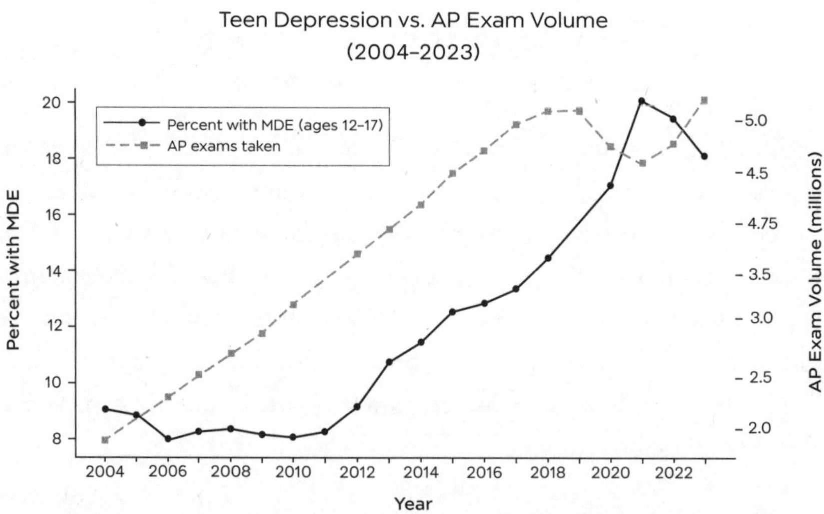

While this curve is not as tight as those for the applications graph above, a clear rise in AP tests over time (with a COVID dip when disruptions to education affected many students) is evident.

Achievement culture and pressure to stand out are being fueled in part by a marked increase in the number of applications to, and the selectivity of, elite colleges. The resultant sense of scarcity created then fuels a further increase in applications and selectivity in what has become a toxic cycle. Let's look now at depression (solid line) with annual numbers of applications since 2004 to Harvard (dashed line) and Stanford (dotted line), two of the most highly selective universities.

Teen Depression vs. Harvard & Stanford Applications (2004–2023)

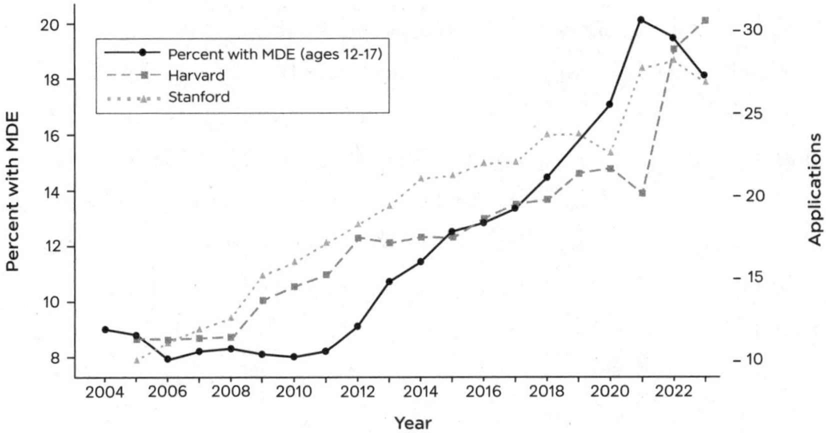

The annual application numbers track closely with the depression rates.

Finally, here is a graph that shows the number of applicants per admitted student at Harvard (dashed line) and Stanford (dotted line) alongside the teen depression rate (solid line).[9, 10, 11] You can see that the number of applicants vying for each coveted spot at Stanford has risen from about eight in 2005, to fifteen in 2015, to about twenty-five in 2022—meaning that it has become increasingly difficult to gain admission.

Teen Depression vs. Applicant-to-Admitted Ratio (Harvard & Stanford), 2004–2023

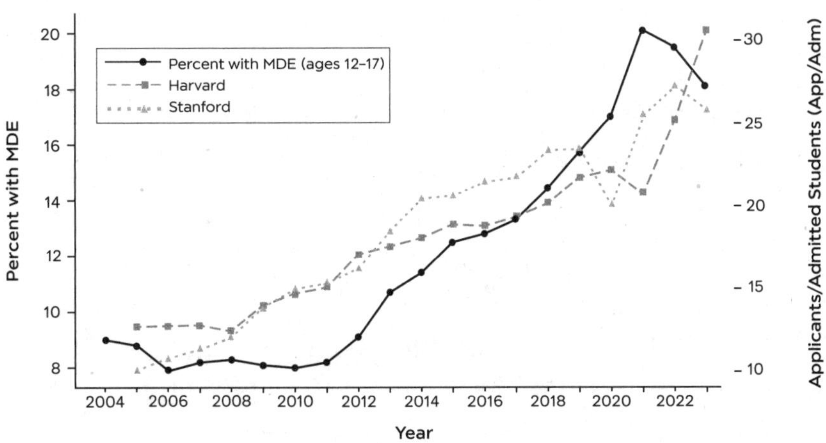

As the number of applicants per spot has soared at these two schools, the number of rejected students has correspondingly skyrocketed. At Stanford that translates into more than fifty thousand students who felt the sting of rejection in 2022, while at Harvard it was close to sixty thousand. And it's not just at the most elite colleges that this is happening. As more and more students apply to multiple schools, they are rejected over and over again. It can be demoralizing, to say the least. In a *New York Times* op-ed titled "We Are the Most Rejected Generation," political and cultural commentator David Brooks explores this barrage of constant rejection experienced by many young people today, who live in a hypercompetitive atmosphere for college, internships, and jobs, and, not surprisingly, he found that it severely affected their sense of belonging, certainty, and self-worth.[12]

As you can see, the data underlying these graphs provide a potential window into how increasing pressure on kids over the past couple of decades tracks with a rise in teen mental illness, a trend that I have documented (as I'll show below) in my research in high schools. At the very least, I hope the graphs have demonstrated to you that there are factors other than digital technology in our teenagers' lives that could be contributing to their increased mental distress. And, as I'll discuss later in the chapter, none of us exist in silos. Teens caught up in the intensity of achievement culture are also buffeted by the pervasive winds of social media; and together they can make for a toxic mix.

My Research into Teen Stress and Distress

Sometimes we forget that real people exist behind the data on a graph or within scientific studies, that for each teen within the "depression cohort," there is a young person struggling, perhaps, to find a sense of self-worth or a modicum of meaning or joy in their life. As a pediatrician, I've cared for thousands of children and teens over the years, so when I decided to do research into the mental health of high schoolers, it made sense to me to engage with the students themselves: to ask them about their lives and what was causing them stress. I believed that when they were asked, they would answer truthfully, providing a window into how they were *really* doing. My aim in doing my research studies was not, like that of many academics, to publish scientific literature. Rather, my goal was to gather information that could help the schools and the kids in them, to shed light on existing problems, and to provide insight into potential targeted interventions that could improve student mental health at those specific schools.

I conducted my first study in 2014 in a high school in the East Bay of San Francisco. Vicki Abeles, the director of *Race to Nowhere,* a widely acclaimed documentary film about the overstressed lives of high school students, connected me to a passionate teacher there, Jay Jackson, and Jay somehow got me through the door. I followed that study with seventeen more, starting with a Catholic girls' school in Missouri, then a school district in the Silicon Valley area, and most recently schools in suburban Ohio in collaboration with two extraordinary nonprofit organizations, MindPeace and 1N5. These communities were not the most affluent—median incomes for the schools were probably in the top 30 percent in the nation; overall, they could be characterized as upper middle class, though with a fairly wide range of family incomes. They were the kind of communities that can be found around any average-sized city in the U.S., the type that parents of young kids gravitate to because of their "good schools." The teens I met with seemed quintessentially American in their own ways. The California kids tended to have a quiet intensity and were open about their desires to attend Stanford, UC Berkeley, or UCLA, while the kids in Ohio with significant college aspirations were less narrowly focused on their future schools and shared more freely the struggles they were experiencing. All were curious and grateful that a pediatrician from St. Louis was concerned about their well-being and was conducting a survey of their mental health.

Surveys

The studies that I led in schools were in many ways very simple in design. The surveys were completely anonymous and were given to kids in the ninth through twelfth grades. While students could opt out of completing them if they wanted to, response rates tended to be very high overall because the kids were given time to complete them in class. They included the following components:

- Questions rating the degree of stress and distress that students were feeling due to a range of factors in their lives
- Estimates of how much time students spent in various activities, including homework, studying, extracurricular activities, and sleep
- Well-accepted and validated depression and anxiety measures (with questions about depression and anxiety symptoms)
- Assessments of problematic mindsets such as maladaptive perfectionism and toxic comparison

I designed the scale for rating stressors in students' lives with the help of many others—educators, mental health experts, researchers, and teens themselves—because I wanted to be sure we captured the range of what might be going on in their lives. Each survey asked the question "To what degree have you felt stressed and/or distressed by each of the following **over the last month**?" (emphasis included in the survey). A list of thirty-five factors followed for students to rate on a five-point scale ranging from 0 (Not at all) to 4 (A great deal). They included those related to school demands (e.g., amount of homework, amount of material I need to learn); school pressure (e.g., pressure from teachers, parent[s], coaches, self); home life (e.g., relationship with parent[s], financial stress); health (e.g., illness/mental illness of a family member; their own health); and social factors (e.g., boyfriend/girlfriend issues, friends, bullying, cyberbullying, and social media). In March of 2021, in the midst of the COVID-19 pandemic, we also asked about fear that they, or a family member, would get sick from COVID.

Ranking of Stressors

At every single high school, we found that the top twelve stressors identified by the teens were all related to school demands and achievement pressure. The order varied slightly in each school, but these were the most common stressors in a rough rank order:

- Pressure from self
- Time pressure
- Pressure to get into a good college
- Pressure not to disappoint your parent(s)
- Fear of failing an exam
- Amount of homework
- Amount of material I need to learn
- Fear of failing a course
- Pressure from parents about school and grades
- Fear of not getting all A's
- Not enough time to spend with my friends
- Pressure to keep up with peers

Cyberbullying and bullying, two issues that have received a fair amount of media attention, often in the aftermath of a suicide, were not rated overall as a big source of stress/distress, ranking thirtieth or lower. It did not mean that there was no bullying or cyberbullying for some individual students, but at a population level, most kids were either not experiencing it or not distressed by it. And what about a student's fears, during a worldwide pandemic in which millions had died, that they or a family member might get sick from COVID? They didn't even crack the top fifteen, logging in respectively as the twenty-fourth and sixteenth most stress-inducing factors.

Time Spent on Homework and Extracurriculars

As part of the survey, students were asked to estimate how much time they spent in various extracurricular pursuits throughout their day. Across all the schools, they reported an average of five hours on weeknights of homework, studying, and extracurricular activities. That was the mean score, so a large number of students were devoting *more* than five hours per day to those activities—in addition to their school day. When I talk to parents during my travels, almost all of them say that these numbers sound right, and as they do so, they usually shake their heads or tell me how absurd or upsetting they find it. "They spend more time working than I do!" is a frequent refrain I hear. The exceptions to the rule are the parents of kids who have opted out and are engaged in their own form of quiet (or not-so-quiet) quitting—though some of them add that these long hours used to be the norm for their child.

Parents and the Pressure to Achieve

Parental pressure was another significant stressor in all the schools I studied. Interestingly, pressure to not disappoint parents was consistently rated as more stressful than pressure *from* parents. It's important to bear in mind that even though you may be a "cool" parent who tells your child not to worry about grades, that their effort and what they're learning are what matters, your kids are likely to notice your overall values. Particularly if you are successful professionals of some kind, your kids will likely feel implicitly that they have to live up to the high bar you have set.

Lack of Sleep

At every single school I studied, kids reported getting about six and a half hours of sleep per night on weekdays on average, a profound sleep deficit for teenagers who should be getting eight to ten hours nightly[13] and a likely contributor to mental health issues (and more), as I will explore and expand upon in chapter 9. Many parents have told me of the continual struggles they have with their teenagers to get them to go to sleep at a reasonable hour, and they often recount that it is a losing battle where they give up and end up going to bed first. Their teens tend to be up, not because they are engaged on their devices, but rather because they are doing homework, finishing a paper, or getting ready for an exam, though, of course, the two can coincide, extending homework hours and pushing back bedtimes.

Maladaptive Perfectionism and Other Problematic Mindsets

One especially interesting—and concerning—finding from the surveys was the prevalence of problematic mindsets in teens in every school. These mental models, or mental filters, shape their views of themselves and their worlds. One of the most distressing is maladaptive perfectionism. It was especially prevalent in my surveys and shows up as kids beating up on themselves repeatedly because of self-perceptions of inadequate performance. I spoke with many students who told me of the profound distress they felt on getting an A minus, their own internal voices screaming *"You're so stupid! You're never going to get into a good college now!"* I also found that many kids reported significant feelings of inadequacy, embarrassment, or shame. You can imagine how some kids feel when they equate self-worth with academic perfection, so that a less-than-stellar grade, or a college rejection, validates their low self-esteem and sends them into despair. In chapter 5, I'll tell you about these mindsets, how they contribute to the "pressure from self" that so many students are experiencing, and their correlations with, and potential contributions to, poor mental health. I will also offer solutions for navigating them.

My research confirmed for me that achievement culture plays a huge role in shaping the lives of high schoolers and affecting their well-being. As you'll see in later chapters, the teens in the schools I surveyed turned out to have significantly high rates of mental illness. For me, the connection between the two is clear. We are creating an unhealthy environment that is harming our kids. No doubt some people will say that my studies have limitations, and I'm well aware of these. First, the responses are all self-report and are therefore susceptible to a range of recall biases. Each of the studies individually involves fairly small populations in communities that are upper middle class and higher, and generalizability to all other communities in the U.S., particularly less-resourced ones, cannot and should not be made. The threats to well-being and mental health may be quite different in communities with different demographics. However, the consistency of findings across the eighteen schools supports the idea that these conditions and problems are real and warrant further investigation, and that they are not limited to the highly affluent communities in big cities on the coasts, as was previously thought.

Just as my research in high schools revealed thousands upon thousands of teenagers struggling under the weight of excessive academic demands that have been normalized, my conversations with parents, educators, counselors, school nurses, and kids themselves showed the same concerns—in Illinois, Minnesota, Ohio, Washington, New York, Massachusetts, Louisiana, Tennessee, North Carolina, and other states, and around the globe in the U.K., France, Switzerland, Singapore, the Netherlands, Taiwan, and Saudi Arabia. In each of these places, I hear a constant refrain about the negative impacts of academic pressure and the overscheduling of kids' lives.

And it's not just teens who are struggling. Recently, a mom told me about her eight-year-old daughter Olivia, a third grader in a public charter school in the city of St. Louis who lives in a virtually continuous anxious state brought on by school demands. The state achievement tests that her teachers tell her will determine where she goes to high school cause her significant distress and confusion. The school ramps up the pressure while telling students there is no need to be anxious. Olivia has said to her mom, "I don't know what I'm supposed to feel!" which only adds to her worry. Before the exam, she is unable to sleep, gets sweaty palms, and shows visible signs of upset, holding a pinched expression on her small face. Throughout the school year, when she doesn't get a perfect score on assignments or tests, she is devastated. There is no gray area, no "I did okay," rather, it's meltdowns with sobs and degrading self-talk: *How could I have done this? How stupid I am!* Her mom has told me how hard it is to witness her daughter's pain. Olivia is a straight-A student; her parents don't put pressure on her; she doesn't have a phone and is not on social media. She is not alone in navigating high anxiety in the face of academic demands; parent after parent has shared with me similar stories of the distress and torment they see in their kids, often long before they reach high school.

Other Research Supporting an Association Between School Pressure and Teen Mental Health

Other research supports my thesis that academic pressure in high school and achievement culture in general contribute to poor mental health among adolescents. Some of the most intriguing research on the subject was done by Dr. Suniya Luthar in the late 1990s and early 2000s, long before the rise in digital technology and screen-based childhoods. Dr. Luthar was studying mental health issues and substance use in tenth graders in under-resourced urban communities, and, needing a control group to compare outcomes, she selected kids in affluent suburban areas. She was stunned by her findings. The kids in the wealthier communities had higher rates of anxiety, depression, and substance use than their less affluent peers who contended with poverty, racism, lack of material resources, and exposure to community violence.[14] The girls from affluent areas had *three times* the rate of depression of those in the general population, while girls and boys had anxiety rates above those of both the general population and the disadvantaged communities that Luthar studied. Her research also probed the potential sources of stress among the privileged teens, and these were her findings:

achievement pressure (particularly as it pertained to gaining admission at an elite college), excessive academic demands, maladaptive perfectionism, and peer competition. Students felt driven to constantly excel in all areas of their lives. The bulk of Luthar's work was done before 2010, well before the arrival of smartphones and Instagram, TikTok, or Snapchat.

We *know* from the work of Luthar and other researchers that school pressure, chronic stress about workload, parental expectations, and competition with peers are associated with harm. A meta-analysis (a "study of studies") on the link between academic pressure and adolescent mental health problems published in 2023 showed that out of fifty-two studies from across the globe, forty-eight found a positive association with at least one negative mental health outcome, including depression, anxiety, suicidal ideation, suicide attempts, or suicide.[15] The studies covered a wide range of schools, including public and private. A large survey of adolescents in the U.K. showed that school stress had a huge influence on their mental health, and in a U.K. study that looked into adolescent suicides, academic pressure was one of the most reported antecedents in coroner investigations.[16] The association between school pressure and a decline in mental health has also been documented in books such as *Doing School: How We Are Creating a Generation of Stressed-Out, Materialistic, and Miseducated Students,*[17] by Denise Pope, and *The Price of Privilege: How Parental Pressure and Material Advantage Are Creating a Generation of Disconnected and Unhappy Kids,*[18] by Madeline Levine.

If these conditions have, as I believe, spread far and wide, then that spread is virtually certain to have contributed to the rise in depression and anxiety seen in the U.S. (and elsewhere) in recent years. If environmental conditions that previously existed largely in the most affluent (say top 10 percent of incomes) have spread to the upper middle class (say the top 30 percent, like the communities where I conducted my research), then three times the number of kids would be affected, thus causing a huge shift in rates of mental illness. If it has spread further, into the upper reaches of the middle class (the top 50 percent of incomes), then five times the number of kids would be affected. Evidence exists that this spread is real.

National surveys of more than 270,000 students conducted by Challenge Success, a school reform program started by Stanford University, have found that students across all income levels report high stress from homework loads, standardized testing, and college admissions expectations.[19] Another piece of evidence to support this spread is the rise of "intensive parenting" across all social classes found in a national study of more than 3,600 parents in 2019. This style of parenting, formerly practiced largely in affluent families, includes prioritization of extracurricular activities such as sports and the visual and performing arts, educational enrichment such as tutoring and educational programs, and time-intensive engagement by parents in kids' activities. The study found that this intensive, child-centered parenting is now pervasive.[20]

Suicide and Suicide Attempts Peak During the School Year

Another lens with which to view links between school/academic pressure and poor mental health in teens is suicide and suicide attempts. Among adults in the U.S. and around the globe, they peak in late spring to early summer. This contrasts with a number of studies of teen suicides that show suicides peaking in the fall and dropping in the summer. One paper from the National Bureau of Economic Research showed that suicide rates were highest during the school year and lowest in the summer months.[21] Strikingly, it also reported that schools that started in August had increases during that month, while those starting in September did not see rises until September. Finally, the researchers found that this pattern changed dramatically in 2020 with school closures during the pandemic. As this report made explicit, "Teen suicides plummeted in March 2020, when the COVID-19 pandemic began in the U.S. and remained low throughout the summer before rising in Fall 2020, when many K-12 schools returned to in-person instruction."

Another recent study concluded, "For Americans ages 15 to 24, the highest spike in suicides was in autumn, September–October, with a trough in June. *This is the only age group in which this occurred* [emphasis mine], differing from a previous understanding of the seasonality of suicide in the literature. With all other age groups (25–34, 35–44, 45–54, 55–64, 65–74, 75+), there was a consistent pattern of a peak in late spring/early summer, a small peak in fall, and a trough in late winter."[22]

Not only do teen suicides peak during the school year and drop during the summer vacation, but, unsurprisingly, psychiatric emergency visits do as well, giving us further insight into the connection between school and poor mental health. A 2023 report from the Centers for Disease Control and Prevention (CDC) found that between 2018 and 2023, visits to emergency departments for depressive disorders, suicidal ideation, and self-harm among kids ages ten to seventeen increased during the fall and spring semesters and fell during the summer, as shown in the figure below.[23]

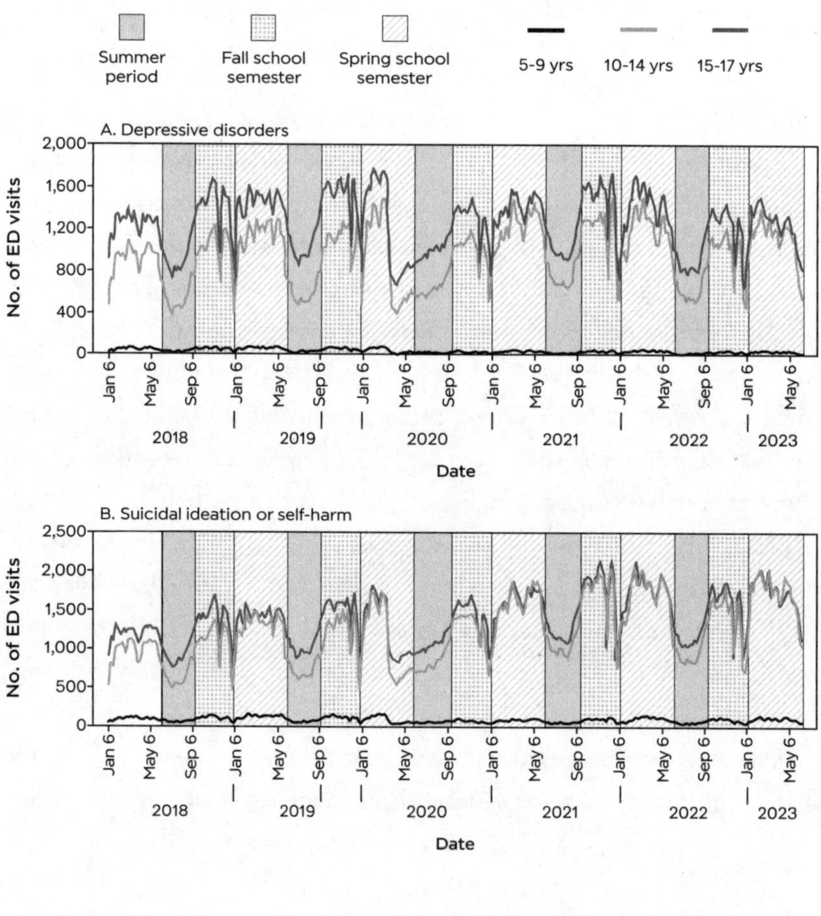

Hospital admissions for psychiatric conditions have also been shown to increase during the school year and decrease in the summer.[24] One final study further supports the school and mental illness connection. A study of schoolchildren in Japan ages eight to twelve found a rise in suicide between 2009 and 2023, with the peak incidence in recent years occurring from April to June.[25] What happens in Japan in April? Unlike in the U.S., that's when the new school year begins.

I'm curious as to what proponents of the tech/social media theory might say about these studies. Use of digital technology varies by time of year, with increased usage during the summer, when kids have more discretionary time, less parental supervision, and later bedtimes.[26] If digital technology is the main driver of mental illness, it might stand to reason that mental illness would peak in the summer as well, yet it clearly doesn't.

These research studies are supported by corroborating stories that I hear from parents. Bella, a bright fifteen-year-old girl, struggles with depression and is treated with antidepressants. In the fall of ninth grade, she started the school year with enthusiasm, but by November she was finding it hard to make it to class. Her attendance remained sporadic throughout the year, and as she fell further behind in her schoolwork, her distress grew and her parents worried that she was suicidal. The summer break couldn't come soon enough. In July, Bella started work at a local animal shelter, arriving early each day, ready to care for the abandoned dogs and cats. Her depression seemed to vanish. But when she returned to school in the fall, she soon felt overwhelmed by the demands of the hectic school day and her depression returned.

Overscheduled Childhoods

As I've spoken with parents across the country about the unremitting pressure that their children face in the quest for high grades, a perfect GPA, and stellar report cards, they also tell me about a massive increase in the number and intensity of extracurricular endeavors that seems to go hand in hand with this pursuit of academic excellence. High schoolers often go straight from school to varsity teams sports practice five days a week, not making it home until 7:00 p.m., or they have dance or play rehearsals, or band practice. Often they are hoping to embellish their résumés and college applications. Parents have reported that these structured activities intrude into our kids' lives at earlier and earlier ages. Six-year-old twin girls who have dance three afternoons a week, swimming lessons on another day, and art class on another. A nine-year-old boy whose baseball practices, games, and travel consume as much as twenty-five hours per week, leaving no time to just hang with friends. Haidt's assessment that free play has largely disappeared from childhood is one that I agree with wholeheartedly. It prevents kids from having time to just be, to experience boredom, follow their curiosity, and enjoy in-person friendships. While he places the blame on two main factors, what he refers to as "experience blockers," which decrease time spent in unsupervised play—the intrusion of screen-based activities and overprotective parenting—I see relentless overscheduling as the primary problem. It's fair to say, however, that we are aligned in our belief that a lack of free play, or downtime, has negative impacts on children's and teens' mental health.

In chapter 9, I'll dive deeply into these so-called enrichment activities, sports, and tutoring and test prep. These activities have all grown in recent years, but the ones that have taken off most and consume ever-growing parts of kids' (and parents') days (and evenings and weekends) are the various club sports. Their daily demands and ever-longer seasons account for a huge time commitment, and the pressures to participate and excel are enormous. What may have started as a love of soccer or swimming is soon turned into another source of competition and stress, and can stretch thin even the most resilient teen who must juggle school and homework with sports practice and meets, squeezing out any time they might have for themselves, for family, or just for hanging out with friends and being a teen. The drive on the part of parents to get their kids engaged in all of these varied activities stems, I believe, largely from fear—from the belief that if you don't offer your kids a full gamut of enrichment opportunities, they won't have a chance of standing out in ways that will get them into the best possible school, high school, or college and enable them to experience success in life.

The One-Two Punch of Social Media and Achievement Pressure

I've made clear throughout this chapter that smartphones and social media *are* a problem, just not the *only* problem when it comes to mental health and kids. This is especially evident when social media and achievement culture collide. Academic pressure and the drive for success don't exist in a vacuum. Instead, when teens ace a test or get into a coveted college, they turn to their socials and let everyone know. Accepted by an Ivy? A celebration video of you opening the email surrounded by family in full college-branded apparel is the perfect way to make the announcement. Apply to twenty colleges with a 4.5 GPA and a strong SAT score and get rejected by eighteen? Then post a video on TikTok chronicling your acceptances and rejections alongside the schools' admissions rates. When social media meets achievement culture, it can amplify constant comparison and cause teens to experience even more stress and anxiety, feel inadequate, and ratchet up the demands and expectations they place on themselves. It can exacerbate an already intense and difficult experience. In many of the schools I surveyed, students spoke to me about the intense pressure they felt to keep up with their peers as well as their fear of being put down by them on social media, often about their academic performance, and the way it filled them with dread. Grades, exam results, and college acceptances or rejections, once private, were now available for public consumption—by friends, peers, family, and complete strangers. It was impossible for them to get away from the ever-intensifying pressure at school, at home, and online—and it was harming their mental health.

• • •

In the next two chapters, I will delve into depression and anxiety, the two most prevalent mental health conditions experienced by kids and teens. I'll share common misconceptions with you, offer thoughts on how you can recognize symptoms and best support your child, and reiterate the need to focus on the role played by achievement culture. The remainder of the book will address another important goal—the steps we can take to prevent kids from ever developing these mental health conditions.

Chapter 2

Depression in the Age of Pressure: What Every Parent Should Know

I conducted my first study of high school students in the East Bay in Northern California. The school was situated in one of a string of suburbs that sprawl along the busy 880 freeway, home to a significant Asian-American population, including large communities of residents of Chinese, Indian, and Filipino descent. Many of the students that I surveyed were first-generation American and spoke to me of the high demands that their school placed on them, as well as heavy pressure from their parents to excel. One boy told me he had cracked under the pressure of elementary school, when he "was just a little egg," and the image stayed with me. It perhaps didn't help the kids that they lived so close to Stanford and UC Berkeley, prestigious colleges that were always on their radar, potential prizes if they could just keep a perfect GPA, score high enough on their SATs, and succeed in a variety of after-school activities. The teens were curious about my research, and I was interested to learn about the stressors they faced and how these affected their lives.

When the results of the survey came in, I was shocked. A stunning 54 percent of the students at the school screened positive for moderate to severe symptoms of depression. My coresearcher, Dr. John Chibnall, who oversaw the statistical analysis for the study, told me that he had run the numbers three times because he just couldn't believe what he was seeing. We had included a well-validated and widely used screen for depression.[1] It consisted of twenty questions, and students could respond on a four-point scale about the frequency of symptoms they were experiencing, from rarely or none of the time to most or all of the time. Symptoms included crying spells, feeling down, and feeling as if everything you do is an effort. Anything from moderate symptoms upward is cause for concern and is generally accepted as defining the approximate depression rate in a population.[2] It was hard to believe that so many of the kids were struggling. I remembered the way they had spilled out of their classes into the California sunshine in their school's outdoor hallways, their energy levels rising. But when we looked at the surveys, we saw that kid after kid had identified their primary stressors as pressure—to get into a good college, to keep up with their peers, to get through an inordinate amount of schoolwork, to maintain an A average, to not disappoint their parents, to not fail exams or courses, to live up to their own expectations.

It was an important lesson for me that kids tend to mask their suffering—or, perhaps, that they thought it was normal to struggle as they were doing. After all, this kind of pressure was all they'd ever known. Whatever the reason, it was clear that without measuring depression in a population of teens and asking kids about their life experiences, you wouldn't know how widespread a problem it is. In small group meetings after taking the survey, students opened up to me and shared their stories. Jason, a tenth grader at the school, told me with downcast eyes that his life was a relentless grind of school, homework, test prep, tutoring, and participation in clubs like Model UN that he wasn't particularly interested in but that were designed to fill out his résumé. He had stopped spending any spare time with friends, preferring to sleep instead. When he shared his concern with his parents that he felt stressed and overwhelmed, they responded with reassurance: "Everyone feels stressed sometimes; you're just tired. You need to be strong!"

I soon discovered that my survey findings were not unique to that Bay Area school and community. Next I surveyed students in a Catholic girls' school in Missouri and found very similar results: survey answers that spoke volumes about kids weighed down by an enormous academic load, with 43 percent of students having moderate to severe symptoms of depression—not quite as high as the California school but still alarming. Since then I have studied sixteen more high schools, and all had depression rates of at least 34 percent. To put this in perspective, a meta-analysis study that looked at fifty-four research studies estimated that the depression rate in medical students—another population affected by academic pressure, long hours, and extremely high expectations—was 27 percent.[3] Another similar study of medical residents estimated a rate of 28 percent.[4] These numbers generated significant alarm within the medical education community, and action was taken to address this issue. By contrast, the depression rates in the high schools I studied garnered attention and concern from teachers and administrators but led to little in the way of serious action to reduce the academic demands and pressure that lay at the heart of the problem.

And that's part of the dilemma. When we hear that teens and students have high rates of depression, we probably have an idea in mind that they have an illness that makes them sad or down some or all of the time, and that medication and talk therapy will likely help them feel better. We think of depression as a problem to be addressed only at the individual level, navigated by the kid, their family, doctors, therapists, and psychiatrists. For the students at the schools I surveyed and for countless others whose parents I've met across the country, depression is often seen as something of a personal failing, one that sidelines some students while others continue to seemingly thrive. We rarely think about the pressure-cooker environment of schools as part of the equation—but this is a mistake.

Evidence that we will dive into throughout the book clearly shows that academic pressure and expectations are associated with depression in adolescents. Given the demands of schools and achievement culture across the country and around the world today, it is likely that many teenagers are at risk of developing depression—or already have it. In this chapter, I'm going to get beyond the misconceptions and inaccuracies to enable you to understand the picture of depression more fully, what it is (and isn't), how it can be caused by your environment, what you can do about it, and how to attend to its root causes—so that you can help the teens and preteens in your life, as they are unlikely to be able to handle it by themselves.

The Role of the Environment in Depression

If your child is diagnosed with depression, it's likely that their doctor or mental health practitioner will be referring to major depressive disorder (MDD), a term that was adopted by the *Diagnostic and Statistical Manual of Mental Disorders* (*DSM*) in 1980. This diagnostic manual, first published by the American Psychiatric Association in 1952, is now in its fifth edition and serves as a classification system for mental health disorders.[5] It sets criteria for healthcare professionals to make various psychiatric diagnoses, including depression. For major depressive disorder, the specific diagnostic criteria must include five (or more) of various symptoms that have been present for a two-week period and represent a change from previous functioning. At least one symptom must be either depressed mood or loss of interest or pleasure, though in children/teens depressed mood can be replaced by irritable mood. Other symptoms include weight loss or gain, changes in appetite, insomnia, fatigue, feelings of worthlessness, difficulty with focus, thoughts of death, or suicidal ideation.

If your child's symptoms meet the criteria, they will be diagnosed with depression, and the focus will generally turn toward treatment rather than identification of the potential underlying cause(s). This is an understandable approach—it's important to help your child feel better—but it is not entirely helpful. Depression has historically been broken down into two main categories based on cause. The first is endogenous, also known as primary depression, which is largely biochemical in nature. It can present suddenly with no precipitating event, is thought of as arising from brain chemistry imbalances involving neurotransmitters such as serotonin and dopamine, and often has a genetic basis, meaning that risk is inherited.

However, not all cases of major depressive disorder are endogenous. Some are known as reactive, situational, or secondary, meaning that they are precipitated by a life event or circumstances such as divorce, death of a loved one, or other trauma; a challenging medical condition; or, especially important for this discussion, excessive stress—as may be found in our kids' highly pressured lives. The lines that differentiate endogenous from reactive depression are not as clear as I just made them sound, and these terms have been abandoned by many modern psychiatrists. In particular, it is simplistic to think of primary depression as purely biochemical, for the individual's situation can have a significant impact on those with primary depression: In other words, a person with endogenous depression in a distressing situation will likely become more depressed. Similarly, there can be biological contributors to reactive depression, including inherited predispositions for it. However, the key takeaway here is that depression can be precipitated by life stressors, including academic and extracurricular pressure.

As I detailed in chapter 1, depression rates in U.S. teens have been rising for some time, with an explosion in cases in recent years. In 2023, the Centers for Disease Control and Prevention (CDC) found in a survey of teens that 40 percent reported experiencing persistent feelings of sadness or hopelessness, 20 percent had seriously considered suicide, and a stunning 9 percent reported that they had attempted suicide—all are associated with depression.[6] There is no reason to believe that our biology, the biochemistry of our brains, has changed drastically over such a short span of time, leading to a spate of new cases of endogenous depression. Therefore, it is much more likely that the vast majority of the rise in depression *must be reactive depression*—in other words, emotional responses to the environment. For many teens, including the thousands who responded to my surveys, the main drivers of this virtually unprecedented prevalence of depression appear to be their highly pressured lives, both in school and in after-school activities. Relentless academic demands and overscheduled days inherent to achievement culture have created a long-term toxic environment that is harmful to their mental health.

How Does This Relate to You?

As a parent, or someone involved in the lives of teens, what can you do with this information? First and foremost, if you have a child who has suffered (or suffers) from depression, and you have felt (or been made to feel) that the problem was with your child, or that they had an illness caused by a chemical imbalance, it may not have been so at all. The truth is that for many teens diagnosed with depression, the problem lies in what school pressure, extracurricular demands, and achievement culture are doing to them. If your child is currently in school, particularly a high-achieving one, then it's important for you to be aware that they are at risk for developing depression. It's not the case for every child or pertinent to every school, but given the intense and stressful environments of many modern schools, parents must be aware that depression is a possibility.

Recognizing Depression: How Does It Manifest in Kids/Teens?

There's a saying in pediatrics that kids are not little adults, and this maxim holds true for depression, as it may not show up in teens in the same way it does in adults. Generally, depression in adults is characterized by low mood, sadness, sleep issues, tiredness, difficulty finding enjoyment in activities, changes in appetite, and weight loss or gain. Sometimes these symptoms may occur in adolescents (so be on the lookout for them), but often teens have very different signs of depression. From the 1960s to the 1980s, symptoms that obscured an underlying depressive disorder were often referred to as "masked depression." The term fell out of favor, probably because of its vagueness and lack of diagnostic precision, but I think it's fairly accurate in describing how parents of teens and health care professionals can easily miss signs of depression because they may look like something else. I encountered various atypical symptoms regularly over the years in my pediatric clinical practice, and I believe it's important to describe or "unmask" them so that you are better able to recognize signs of depression in a child you care about. These atypical symptoms tend to fall into four main categories: somatic, cognitive, social, and behavioral.

Somatic (Bodily) Complaints

In my practice, somatic complaints were the symptoms I most frequently encountered. These included headaches and chest pain (the most common of the pain sites, in my experience), but also body aches, stomach pain, fatigue, and low energy. When I would see a teenager with recurrent episodes of chest pain in the clinic at UCLA, I often asked the resident or medical student I was working with to estimate how often a heart or lung problem would be the cause of this presenting symptom. They tended to be strongly biased in their thinking, believing that some kind of physical ailment would be likely. None of them came close to what my experience was, which was *never.*[7] It isn't that a teen with recurrent episodic chest pain cannot have some type of nonpsychological cause, but I had seen dozens of patients with this problem over my twenty-one years of pediatric experience, and not one of them had a physical cause—not a single one. Generally speaking, kids that age almost never suffer from ailments such as coronary artery disease, which would cause angina (cardiac chest pain). But huge numbers of them were experiencing significant life stressors—family, school, and social—and their pain was a direct manifestation of that. Despite this, I always did a careful history and physical exam to ensure that I wasn't encountering my first cardiac, or other physical, cause. An unwritten law of good medical practice is: Look for psychosocial causes of physical symptoms, but don't leap too quickly to that diagnosis. It's important to point out that chest pain and other somatic symptoms not only are associated with depression but also can be signs of chronic stress (of all kinds), anxiety, PTSD, or grief. So, the more crucial tasks for me were to interview the teen and the parents to try to determine what could be the underlying psychosocial source(s) of the pain, identify the most likely psychiatric diagnosis if they had one, and refer them for mental health care if indicated.

Cognitive Symptoms

It is not uncommon to see cognitive symptoms, including poor concentration, difficulty focusing, forgetfulness, and distractibility, in depressed teens. These can be accompanied by declines in grades and increasing apathy, in a self-perpetuating cycle that typically includes persistent self-criticism, a relentless focus on perceived personal inadequacies, hopelessness, and a sense of failure. Jason, our stressed and overwhelmed tenth grader with likely depression, told me that he had difficulty concentrating in the evenings when he was doing his homework and that while his grades had not suffered, the extra time needed to complete his work had led him to get less and less sleep, leaving him even more exhausted.

Social Symptoms

Social behaviors related to depression (other than those described in the behavioral issues outlined below) tend to be characterized by some form of withdrawal and/or isolation. Teens may lose interest in activities they used to enjoy, reduce participation in outside activities such as sports or hobbies, try to avoid or minimize social interactions, and/or retreat to their rooms for excessive, and increasingly longer, periods of time. Any efforts made by parents or siblings to encourage more engagement or less isolation are generally met with resistance by the teen. In one case, I saw a twelve-year-old girl who was brought in by her parents because of her progressive withdrawal from family and friends. When I talked to her without her parents in the room (something I always did during teen checkups), she cried as she told me how stressed she felt, said she didn't want to go to school any more, and said her parents repeatedly chastised her if she received a score of less than 100 on exams or assignments. Another teen admitted that he felt stupid around his friends, who all did better in school than he did, and so he no longer wanted to hang out with them.

Behavioral Symptoms

A wide range of problematic behaviors can be seen with depression in teens, including irritability, short temper and outbursts of anger, oppositional behaviors, frequent arguments, hostility, risk-taking, and substance use. As a pediatrician, when I saw this profile in teens, it was important to not just think of them as "difficult" kids and simply guide parents around issues such as rules, limits, and consequences. Rather, it was critical to try to determine whether these behaviors were associated with some significant life stressor—which was often the case—and identify what that was and seek ways to help the family understand and manage that dynamic. In one case, a family brought their teen son in to see me because of episodes of rage, cursing, and flouting of household rules. When I spoke with the teen alone, he broke down and cried as he shared that his father was placing huge pressure on him in baseball, pushing him to practice all the time, criticizing him when his performance was lacking, and berating him if he made an error in a game. He described difficulty sleeping and poor appetite, and I referred him to our child and adolescent psychiatrists for evaluation for possible depression. I also spoke gently with the parents about my concern that the pressure that was being placed on their son in baseball could be contributing to his behavior and that a softer approach might be helpful.

It's important to note that these symptoms tend to have different prevalences in males and females. Boys are more likely to engage in what are called *externalizing* behaviors, meaning they are outward-facing. These include rule-breaking, angry, or "aggressive" behaviors, including defiance, risk-taking, and furious expression as opposed to sadness. Girls are more prone to *internalizing* behaviors, such as frequent crying, dwelling on mistakes, cutting/self-harm, rumination, social withdrawal, restrictive eating, and physical symptoms and complaints. One could generalize that boys tend to direct the pain they are feeling out at the world, and girls to direct their pain inward, at themselves. Let me emphasize that these gendered tendencies are just that—these signs can be seen in both genders as well as in nonbinary kids. In recent years, among boys especially, internalizing symptoms have risen while externalizing symptoms have decreased sharply.[8] Jason was an excellent example of this. He wasn't having outbursts or engaging in risk-taking behaviors as many boys with depression do; rather, he had begun to withdraw from his family and his friends, spending more time alone in his room.

What to Do If You Suspect Depression

Take Action

It can be scary to think that your child might have a mental illness, and sometimes you may feel that it's better not to know for sure—but not knowing won't make the symptoms disappear or your kid feel better. You may believe that you don't have time for appointments or that your teen can't take time out from school to attend them. In this situation, it's vital to look at the big picture. If you think your child may be experiencing depression, then getting them help must take priority.

One factor that may prevent action is your own past experience as an adolescent facing demands and pressures; you may feel that you got through it, and your child will too. We have to recognize that many kids are facing pressures today that are *unprecedented* and it isn't appropriate to extrapolate from your own school experience years ago and make assumptions about your child. Another common factor that can lead to inaction is a hope or belief that your teen will grow out of what they're going through. I've known many parents who have entertained the idea that symptoms of depression in adolescence are just a phase that their child will emerge from unscathed. However, depression as a teenager is accompanied by significant potential long-term consequences—primarily, a substantial increase in the likelihood of struggling with depression as an adult. In a systematic review research paper published in 2018, seventeen of eighteen longitudinal studies showed an increased rate of depression in adulthood for those who had depression in adolescence. When results from the studies were pooled, a 2.78-fold increase in depression risk was found—in other words, a depressed adolescent is more than two and a half times more likely to suffer from depression as an adult than teens who are not depressed.[9]

It is better to act sooner rather than later, while your child is under your roof and in your care. After high school, late adolescents/young adults will face new challenges to their mental health. Those jumping directly into the workforce, aspiring to live independently while often earning low wages, face enormous challenges to simply make ends meet, which produces feelings of chronic, persistent stress and threat. If they have health insurance, it is not likely to have expansive mental health benefits, and copays for mental health services may prove to be a huge barrier to receiving care. Even with good coverage, shortages of mental health services may also impede access.

College offers no safe harbor. Stresses are inherent in the transition to college, including new academic and extracurricular demands and pressure, and a new social world to navigate. These challenges are often confronted without the immediate support of family or an encouraging peer group from high school. Access to mental health services is often limited or delayed, and depression among college students is not simply high; it's on the rise. The Healthy Minds Study, a large national survey of college students, found that the prevalence of depression rose from 24 percent to 31 percent between 2013 and 2018.[10] The rates have almost certainly increased since then. Subpopulations in higher education such as STEM majors, premeds, engineering students, and college athletes likely suffer even higher rates. A study I did with Dr. Asmira Alagic and undergraduate student Liz Pfau, published in 2024, screened students in an introductory chemistry course (many of them premed) for depression, in an anonymous survey. We found that 49.3 percent of students screened positive with moderate to severe symptoms of depression.[11]

My recommendation is that if you think your teen or preteen is depressed, find out more, and get them the treatment they need by following the steps below while it is easier for you to help them through the process. Don't let any sense of stigma or shame prevent you from acting—your duty is to your child who needs your full support at this time.

Get an Evaluation

Let me start by emphasizing that if you see some symptoms in your child, it doesn't necessarily mean that they have depression, as there are multiple possible other causes. That's why having a careful, thorough evaluation by a health care professional with significant experience in the care of children is critically important, whether that is a pediatrician, a family physician, an adolescent specialist, or a nurse practitioner. You know your child best, and if something seems "off" to you, or their behavior or demeanor seems to have shifted, trust yourself and seek an evaluation from a professional. You could also consider reaching out to a mental health provider earlier rather than later (you could get a referral from your pediatrician, the school nurse, or your own personal network). It's best if a child is not in crisis before mental health care is sought (though if they are, seeking help is more important than ever).

Treatment Options

If the evaluation indicates that your child has depression, a number of potential treatment options are available. It is unlikely that you will be told the cause of the depression, but the treatment protocol for all depression tends to be the same: talk therapy with or without antidepressant medication. I'll review these options next, but first I'd like to encourage a broadening of our view of the management of depression. Treatment is vitally important, but especially in the case of reactive depression, we would also want to make changes to the environment that is causing it. I offer solutions later in the book to address the stressors in your kids' lives, describing how schools can reduce pressure and demands as well as how parents can make choices in order to avoid adding to the pressure kids are feeling outside the home. These remedies can be used in conjunction with the standard treatment protocols for depression reviewed in this chapter.

Talk therapy: The most common form of talk therapy is cognitive behavioral therapy (CBT). It has been the dominant approach in psychotherapy for many decades and is practiced by a majority of mental health practitioners. It emphasizes the importance of thoughts in changing behaviors and involves developing skills in cognitive restructuring, which comprises noticing, labeling, and disputing the stories we are telling ourselves. I've found that it can be extremely helpful for teens with depression. Other useful therapies include dialectical behavior therapy (DBT) and acceptance and commitment therapy (ACT), which I'll elaborate on in the next chapter since they are the first-line treatments for anxiety as well. All three are evidence-based interventions that focus on helping kids manage their thoughts in ways that render them less harmful, and have been shown to be effective in the treatment of adolescent depression in a number of studies.[12]

Medication: The other path, which can be combined with talk therapy, is antidepressant medication. These medications may be appropriate as treatment and can be helpful for some kids. They can have side effects ranging from dry mouth, headaches, gastrointestinal symptoms, drowsiness, or, conversely, insomnia, to, of most concern, an increase in suicidal thoughts and behaviors in a small percentage of kids. It's important to note that treatment for depression doesn't have to be either/or. Not surprisingly, combining antidepressant medication with talk therapy has been found to be more effective than medication alone.[13]

Relief from symptoms of depression can take time while teens adjust to therapy and/or as the medication kicks in. It's important to be patient. Consistency with therapy sessions is also key. Sometimes parents and teens are eager to stop treatment when they see an improvement in symptoms, but it's best to listen to recommendations from the mental health provider—often more progress can be made as kids are less affected by symptoms.

Suicide

Depression can lead to thoughts of suicide (suicidal ideation) and/or suicide attempts. (Note: Suicidal ideation is multi-factorial and is not always preceded by depression.) Be aware if your child's symptoms seem to get worse, and have a plan in place in case they do. This might be reaching out to their pediatrician or their therapist. If your child appears to be severely depressed and expresses such thoughts as "I wish I were dead, you'd be better off without me," or "I can't take this anymore," or engages in behaviors such as giving away prized possessions or calling people to say "goodbye," then you need to act immediately.

- Ask if they are thinking about hurting themselves (asking about suicide will not put the idea into their head or spur them to action).
- Show them immediate support and concern—and listen without judgment.
- Secure "lethal means" such as firearms, sharp objects, medications (prescribed and over-the-counter), and toxic substances like cleaning supplies.
- Call or text 988, the Suicide and Crisis Lifeline, or text HOME (or AYUDA) to 741741, the Crisis Text Line, for help in navigating the situation.
- Contact a mental health professional as soon as possible.
- Consider taking them to a hospital emergency room for immediate assessment and care.

How to Support Your Child If They Are Depressed

While navigating the health care system is a vital role for parents if your child has depression, it isn't your only role. Another important one is directly supporting your child. There are a whole range of parenting approaches and philosophies that may be helpful—I offer several here and have much more to say on the subject in the coming chapters. These suggestions have not been proven in double-blind, placebo-controlled studies; however, as many parents may agree, they are hard to argue with.

- Believe in your child and make them feel that belief. Tell them that you love them and that you are there for them, no matter what.

- Help them manage any self-critical narratives that they may have. If they say something like "I'm so stupid," try to counter by disagreeing and providing evidence against this negative thought. (Much more on this to come in chapter 5 (on problematic mindsets) and chapter 6 (on cognitive distortions).
- Try not to contribute unnecessarily to the pressure they already feel. For example, try to avoid being overly critical when their performance isn't stellar. Be interested in all aspects of their life, not just how they're doing in their schoolwork.
- Advocate strongly for them when needed, but avoid becoming a constantly hovering parent, or a snowplow parent, relentlessly clearing obstacles in their path. They still have to learn to handle age-appropriate situations, even as they navigate depression.
- Find support for yourself so that your concern for your child doesn't add to their burden. It could be speaking with a trusted family member or friend, your doctor, a spiritual leader, or a mental health practitioner.
- Know that you'll sometimes get things wrong, and try to forgive yourself when you do. Just as importantly, endeavor to learn from your mistakes.
- Don't feel ashamed by your child's struggles in any way or feel as if your child's struggles reflect badly on your family. This may be harder than it sounds.

Shame

It's worth spending some time on the topic of shame and how cultural views can affect parental (and grandparental) attitudes about depression and mental illness. Even though we are moving toward a more accepting and open approach to mental health in general in the U.S., it can still be difficult for parents to accept that their child has a mental health disorder.

They may blame themselves—or their child—for their "failure" and may worry about judgment from other family members, neighbors, or their social and/or school community. Their child's mental health condition can become a big secret—which can have multiple negative repercussions for the teen.

In my over thirty years of experience in medical education, I have come to know thousands of students from multiple cultures. Among these were first-generation Americans from immigrant families, and many of these students shared with me that they could not reveal to their parents that they were depressed or anxious and that they needed or were receiving mental health care.[14] The word that came up again and again in those conversations with these students was *shame,* that having a child with mental illness would bring shame to the parents and upon the entire family. These conversations had a huge emotional impact on me. But let me hasten to add that such an attitude toward mental illness and mental health care is not limited to this, or any, cultural group. I'm happy to say that many of my former students are now parents and have moved far from their own parents' ideas. I hope that beliefs continue to shift, because shame, no matter the culture, is a powerful toxin that too often keeps depression and other forms of mental illness in the dark and can get in the way of much-needed treatment.

Getting to the Root of the Problem

Treatments for depression as outlined above are often effective and can change people's lives. If your teen shows symptoms of depression, I urge you to make sure they get the appropriate care. This is a critical step that can vastly improve the mental health of your child, which is, of course, of paramount importance to you as a parent. The systemic problem—the mental health crisis of teens in America—remains, however, and addressing and alleviating this problem will require a different kind of intervention; we cannot solve the problem if we ignore root causes.

To a great degree, depression has been medicalized—meaning, it is largely seen as a biochemically mediated disease that we need to screen for and then treat. This is not the *only* lens through which depression is viewed, but it is currently the dominant one within the greater American psyche. The U.S. research enterprise has historically been heavily biased toward the biomedical view, which involves understanding chemical pathways, deepening our understanding of the human brain, and testing the safety and efficacy of various pharmaceutical agents. The American Psychiatric Association (APA), the largest professional organization of psychiatrists in the U.S. and a powerful entity in its own right, has tended to focus on pathology and treatment, while paying less attention to identifying root causes that are environmental in nature.

This means that we continue to primarily follow a treatment model for depression in youth, rather than seek ways to prevent it.[15] The American Academy of Pediatrics (AAP), an organization that I have deep admiration and respect for, is one of the leading child health advocacy organizations in the world, and a major focus of their work has been on prevention and health promotion. Over the years, they have held campaigns and developed resources to encourage good nutrition and healthy eating habits, promote physical activity, prevent accidents such as drowning, promote vaccination, reduce screen time, and encourage the use of car seats and seat belts, to name a few. The roster of areas the AAP has touched and illuminated is long and impressive; however, it has not, nor has the U.S. healthcare system more broadly, adequately addressed prevention in the ongoing teen mental health crisis.

The organization *has* recommended universal yearly screens for depression in teens and released two sets of comprehensive guidelines for pediatricians related to depression, which is not insignificant.[16] Each provides robust recommendations for assessing, identifying, and managing kids with depression. But they say nothing about trying to *prevent* the condition. Their recommendations are sound, but what are you going to do when 54 percent of kids in a given population are depressed? Universal screening is a start, but we will never have enough therapists to treat all of the depressed kids—and is that really the answer? We shouldn't simply be treating the symptoms; we should be proactively assessing the environment that we know is a primary contributor to the problem.

The mental health crisis in healthcare workers has been tied directly to the demands and toxicity of the work environment itself. The same is true in the armed services, where suicide rates are markedly high and where high-pressure jobs and frequent deployment are the main foci of presumed causes. The same goes for rising suicides in the college athlete population. In one large study, the authors stated: "Athletes are generally thought of as one of the healthiest populations in our society, yet the pressures of school, internal and external performance expectations, time demands, injury, athletic identity, and physical fatigue can lead to depression, mental health problems, and suicide."[17] In each of these examples above, we have recognized that it's what we are *doing to people* that is the root cause and that it needs to be addressed if we are to bring about change. We need to bring this same thinking to environmental causes of teen depression.

Lessons about addressing root causes of illness can be learned from Flint, Michigan, where, in 2015, people began to notice changes to the taste, smell, and appearance of their drinking water: a metallic tang, a strong and unpleasant aftertaste, a musty sewer-like odor, and a brown, murky discoloration with visible sediment and floating particles. At the same time, pediatricians were hearing parents voice concerns about vague symptoms, such as fussiness and delayed developmental milestones in their kids. It took an extraordinary individual, pediatrician Dr. Mona Hanna (formerly Hanna-Attisha), to connect the dots, to act, and to also push others to act. She had heard concerns from parents about their kids' symptoms and about the water, and a conversation with a friend from high school who worked at the Environmental Protection Agency (EPA) enabled her to put it all together: The drinking water was contaminated with lead and likely causing the symptoms in kids. Dr. Hanna knew how serious this situation could be.

Physical symptoms of lead poisoning can be notoriously mild, vague, and at times even absent, while at the same time those lead levels, if present for long enough, can cause behavioral problems, learning disabilities, and potentially permanent cognitive impairment. Knowing she had to act fast, she reviewed records of blood tests at Hurley Medical Center, where she worked, and found a striking increase in lead levels. She then held a press conference to present her findings that Flint's water was contaminated with lead and that people's health, especially children's, was being harmed. State officials initially scoffed, dismissing her evidence as flawed. She persisted, however. She knew they needed to get the lead out of their water supply to address the community's health issues at the root. Action was taken soon after, with President Obama declaring a federal emergency in Flint in January 2016.

It would have been completely ineffective to manage the Flint kids' symptoms without attending to the lead in the water. A bigger fix was needed. But that is, in effect, what we're doing with the adolescent mental health crisis. To make a difference, we must do more than treat symptoms in individual kids. We need to remediate the source of the problem, to prevent depression and other conditions before they can occur. Just as the kids in Flint would not have gotten better without our addressing the water contamination, depression rates in our country's teens will not improve unless we address the factors contributing to the mental health crisis. What's clear to me and to a multitude of concerned parents is that for far too many communities and kids in this country and around the world, excessive academic demands, achievement culture, and a frenzied pursuit of success are the lead, the toxin, in our kids' environments. But the good news after that ominous sentence is that, just as in Flint, we can do something about it—and I'll provide suggestions for solutions later in the book.

Chapter 3

Understanding Anxiety: When Normal Worry Turns to Distress

Fifteen-year-old Emma was midway through the fall semester of her sophomore year at a public academic magnet school, and her parents were worried that she seemed to be falling apart. Each day began with episodes of sobbing, trembling, and pleas to not send her to school, and they showed no signs of abating.

Transitions to new school years had always been difficult for Emma. She was perpetually the youngest in her grade, her birthday having fallen just within the cutoff for entry into kindergarten, and it still seemed to make an impact. Her parents regretted that they hadn't held her back a year, but she was such a bright and curious child that it seemed a shame to not let her progress from preschool with her friends. Over the past few years, as summer break came to a close, Emma's worry about a return to school invariably began, and her cheerful demeanor slipped away. On the first day of each new school year, she begged her parents to let her stay home, noting that she knew kids who were home-schooled and doing great and *why couldn't she do that?!* There were tears and threats and a refusal to eat breakfast, but then she got in the car because she didn't want to be late on the first day back. As the weeks passed, she seemed to acclimatize to school, enjoying her classes and her friends, her worries returning before tests and then receding . . . until the next school year rolled around.

The start of ninth grade was especially tough. The pressure and demands had amped up compared to middle school, and Emma's perfectionistic tendencies led to late-night studies and diminished sleep, but over time she rallied, as she had each year before. She had a tight circle of friends (mostly girls that she'd known for years) with whom she laughed easily, even if they'd spent more time studying than laughing recently. She stayed at a baseline level of anxiety that seemed acceptable to her mom and dad. After all, they thought, all teens had some level of anxiety, didn't they?

This year was different, though. September had arrived with its usual flurry of stress for Emma, accompanied by sleepless nights, crying sessions, and waves of nausea. On her first day of school, she looked exhausted and tense as she sat in the car, as if she were heading toward her doom. Her parents exchanged glances and hoped that things would settle down as in the past, that the routine and social activities would buoy her. But it didn't happen. Her academic load had increased substantially—there seemed to be a test for every subject every week—and homework was never-ending, and, as Emma complained, often pointless. Volleyball practices stretched longer, with competition for a spot on the team growing more intense. Her friends seemed different too, focused on school, busy all the time, and never wanting to hang out. The worry and anxiety that had always eased in prior years seemed to grow and engulf Emma. She developed muscular tics—brief twitches of her mouth and eyes—that looked like grimaces of pain.

At a visit to her longtime pediatrician, Emma and her parents were reassured that the problem wasn't some neurological disease and that Tourette syndrome was unlikely. However, the pediatrician was concerned and fairly certain that the tics were caused by stress and, given Emma's history, that the source seemed to be the demands and pressures of school. He recommended that she see a therapist, the sooner the better, preferably one who used some form of cognitive behavioral therapy. "The front desk will give you some referrals," he said, before adding, "There's a big demand for mental health services in the community. So be aware that you may have to wait a while for an appointment." He also suggested that they talk to the school to make sure they knew about Emma's struggles—and to ask if the demands could be ratcheted down at all. He had a number of patients in the same school and others in the area like it who seemed to be buckling under the strain.

Over the next few days, Emma's parents left messages with four therapists, then reached out to the high school principal and met with her to share their story and the pediatrician's recommendations. The principal listened with appropriate concern, leaning forward, and offering tissues when Emma's mom grew teary as she and her husband described Emma's state. When they got to the topic of homework and expectations, they expressed their sense that these were excessive and asked if they could be reduced. The principal paused for a moment, then responded gently, "I see parents in my office who want *more* homework. This is an academic magnet school and our focus must be on academics. We have to be competitive. You may want to consider a consultation with a learning specialist. Has Emma ever been evaluated for a learning disability?"

"But she gets straight As. I don't think that could be the issue," said the mom.

"You'd be surprised," said the principal. "They can go unseen for years and appear as a student progresses in school. Maybe Emma needs some tutoring and support."

That same day, Emma's mom called the child development clinic at the local medical center and was informed that a comprehensive evaluation would cost $5,000 and wasn't usually covered by insurance. To make things worse, the next appointment wasn't available for five months—unless someone canceled. Emma's mom was bewildered, but feeling like she didn't have a choice, she had Emma added to the wait list. She still wasn't convinced that this was the right approach, but it felt wrong not to investigate it if it could help her daughter's situation. She wasn't sure where the money would come from, but they would have to figure it out.

Six weeks later, they received a call, asking if Emma could come in the next day for the learning evaluation as a last-minute cancellation had opened up a spot. To the parents, it felt like progress. Emma protested, however, refusing at first to miss school, not wanting to get behind on her work, but she finally acquiesced. If this could improve her academic performance, maybe it would be worth it. Over the next four days, Emma went through a series of assessments, some fifteen hours in all, involving a detailed intake history and a battery of tests with a dizzying array of acronyms: the WISC-V, the WIAT-4, the D-KEFS, and the CPT-3. "Do you think I passed?" Emma asked her mom each day. "What if I didn't? What then?"

A week later, Emma and her parents met with the director of the clinic to receive the report. The results indicated that she didn't have a learning disability. To the contrary, she had excelled in tests of a range of cognitive areas, including executive functioning, verbal comprehension, visual/spatial processing, mathematics, and written comprehension and expression. Emma's parents, her teachers, and Emma herself had completed instruments assessing her for attention-deficit hyperactivity disorder (ADHD) and that had come up negative as well. What the evaluators had found most notable, however, was her very high score on a screen for anxiety—and her repeated nervous questions throughout the testing process of *How am I doing? I'm doing okay, right? I screwed that one up, didn't I? Am I going to fail?*

"To be honest," said the director, "we see this a lot. Very bright kids like Emma at high-achieving schools with significant levels of anxiety. Our recommendation is therapy."

"She has her first appointment next week," said Emma's dad. "It took a while to get one."

"See how it goes," said the director. "Give it some time. But if things don't improve, our other suggestion is to consider changing schools. The pressure is only going to get worse next year."

"No way," said Emma, looking concerned. "I'm not switching. I can't . . . It's the best school. I'll be fine." Even as she spoke, her mouth twitched.

Watching their daughter hunched in her chair, her face contorted in pain, Emma's parents felt overwhelmed. How had it come to this? The academic magnet school they had chosen to support Emma's chances of future success now seemed only to push her farther from that intended goal. Was the school and all it entailed worth it?

Teen Anxiety Rates

There are countless kids like Emma who are experiencing anxiety. The rates of anxiety disorders in teens and young adults are high and on the rise. A study from 2010 by Jean Twenge and colleagues found that anxiety rates in high school and college students had increased steadily over decades.[1] She made the stunning observation that "the birth cohort change in anxiety is so large that by the 1980s normal child samples were scoring higher than child psychiatric patients from the 1950s"—and that was forty years ago, well before the recent dramatic upsurge. The National Survey of Children's Health, which has tracked anxiety rates in teens since 2016, found in 2023 that 16.1 percent of adolescents ages twelve to seventeen had a current diagnosis of an anxiety disorder (which I will define later in this chapter), up from 10 percent in 2016.[2] That's a huge increase in just seven years. Another national survey, the National Comorbidity Survey Adolescent Supplement, found that about a third of teens ages thirteen to eighteen had had an anxiety disorder during their lifetime (meaning in their life to date, though not necessarily at the time of the survey).[3] The college data are also alarming. The American College Health Association has conducted national surveys that include questions about anxiety since 2008. The findings are astonishing. The number of students reporting ever being diagnosed with anxiety has more than tripled, rising from 10.4 percent in 2008 to 34.6 percent in 2022. The percentage of students reporting feeling overwhelming anxiety in the previous two weeks increased from 19.4 to 29.6 between 2008 and 2019.[4]

In the high schools that I studied, a huge number of students were struggling with anxiety.[5] In the school in the East Bay, in Northern California, and the Catholic girls' school in Missouri, the rates were substantially higher than national levels: A remarkable *80 percent* of students in the former school and *84 percent* in the latter had moderate to severe symptoms of anxiety. The chilling takeaway is that there are high schools and communities around the country where anxiety is the *norm* and kids without anxiety are outliers. While my subsequent studies in other high schools did not find rates quite that high, they all exceeded 40 percent—

which is still an unprecedented number of teens struggling under the burden of anxiety.

Research shows that academic pressure is tied to increased anxiety in teenagers. From Luthar's work to more recent studies, we see that these heated school environments can have a detrimental effect on kids' mental health. A systematic review on the association between academic pressure and adolescent mental health problems published in 2023 (and mentioned in chapter 1) looked at five cross-sectional studies that focused solely on academic pressure and anxiety. All five studies found a link between the two.[6] In a narrative review from 2024, the authors examined a range of potential influences on teen anxiety, including individual, familial, societal, and environmental factors, and they concluded that academic pressure was associated with higher anxiety levels.[7] They recommended that further research is needed to understand what interventions may be appropriate to "encourage academic excellence while minimizing undue stress." A 2018 report on adolescent wellness from the Robert Wood Johnson Foundation called attention to school or family pressure as a significant cause for concern, stating, "The challenges youth face when their environments do not foster well-being cannot be ignored. The reality is that some environments make it harder for kids to succeed."[8] Along with poverty, past and current trauma, racism, sexism, homophobia, xenophobia, and other discrimination, the report highlighted "excessive pressure to excel" as one such environment that "can affect youth in significantly deleterious ways, including causing high levels of stress and anxiety or alcohol and drug use and dependence." Excessive pressure to excel succinctly summarizes achievement culture.

Just as with depression, we are failing, or unwilling, to see what is hiding in plain sight. Adolescents are experiencing anxiety at record levels. Research clearly demonstrates the link between academic pressure/achievement culture and anxiety, but instead of looking for ways to address the toxic learning environment and reduce the pressure, we medicalize, or pathologize, anxiety. Anxiety is often viewed as a "disorder," an illness with the problem centered exclusively in the individual. When Emma developed tics and extreme distress in the face of unreasonable academic expectations, her school's reaction was to shift the conversation and suggest that she might have a learning disorder, that her anxiety was an individual problem. To her parents' suggestion that the academic load was unduly heavy, the principal pointed to other parents and to the society we live in that deemed these relentless demands appropriate and necessary. Instead of questioning this narrative, the head implied that Emma's inability to thrive was her issue alone. But when so many millions of teens across the country are experiencing unprecedented levels of anxiety—think of the 80 to 84 percent in two of the high schools I studied and the more than 40 percent in the others—how can this be the case? How can we *not* view their anxiety instead as a largely understandable reaction to an abnormal, excessively stressful environment—one that needs to change?

Currently, as with depression, more attention and resources are directed to screening, diagnosis, and treatment of anxiety than they are to prevention. The American Academy of Child and Adolescent Psychiatry and the American Academy of Pediatrics have collaborated on thoughtful practice guidelines for pediatricians relating to anxiety, and their work helps numerous children; their focus, however, is almost entirely on detection and management. These measures are, of course, crucially important and should continue to be supported so that we can get help to kids who need it. But the fact is that there are simply not enough therapists to handle the deluge of kids, teens, and young adults today who are experiencing debilitating anxiety. Bleaker still is the reality that many of those who are suffering will never access the care they need because of a whole host of reasons, including stigma, lack of insurance or underinsurance, lack of time, cost, obstacles to access, skepticism about efficacy, apathy, and/or hopelessness. We need to work on bringing much-needed awareness to parents of the role that relentless pressure plays in rising anxiety rates in kids and teens, and we need to shift, or rebalance, the focus on what we can do to prevent it.

Emma and her parents are not alone in trying to navigate school-related anxiety. In my work, I've spoken with many families just like them whose lives have been turned upside down by an anxious child's difficulties in schools that refuse to see, let alone acknowledge, that the learning environment itself is contributing to students' deteriorating mental health. Universally, these families have felt unsupported and unheard through much of their journey. In this chapter, I look at anxiety with a view to helping you understand it, recognize it, and know when you should be concerned. I'll suggest some effective ways to support your child if they are struggling. I'll also help you see that recognition and treatment are vitally important *and* that they will never be sufficient to stem the teen anxiety epidemic. We must also address the root causes found in the environment.

Understanding Worry, Normal Anxiety, and Clinical Anxiety

With the increased media and public health spotlight on the teen mental health crisis in general and anxiety in particular, it can be hard to remember that some anxiety is inevitable and even beneficial. I imagine that on seeing the words *normal anxiety* you may even have had the reaction, *What? Anxiety can be normal?* The answer is yes, absolutely—it is an expected and unavoidable reaction to the inevitable stresses in life. As a parent, you need to know what normal anxiety looks like and how it differs from worry and clinical anxiety. Only then can you take the best steps to support your child.

Before we dive into worry, normal anxiety, and clinical anxiety, I need to say a few words about a factor that lies at the heart of all three—stress. One major challenge in clarifying the terms is that the word *stress* is used in several different ways. The first usage involves stress that comes from outside forces. This is external stress (or stressors) and can include small things, such as running late for an appointment or facing a quiz, or large things, such as divorce or a family member with a serious illness. The second common usage of the word *stress* relates to a personal feeling—"I'm feeling stressed." This can be synonymous with being worried or anxious depending on its nature and intensity. The third common usage is the "biological stress response," also known as our fight-or-flight mechanism—

your bodily/physical response to an external stressor. We will delve deeper into this later in the chapter.

Worry

Worry is a cognitive process that involves thoughts that tend to be future focused about perceived problems or threats. For your teen, it could be related to any number of activities or scenarios: an upcoming test, a visit to the dentist, or how many likes they'll get on an Instagram post. Worries tend to be short-lived and don't interfere with one's daily functioning.

Normal Anxiety

Normal anxiety involves the cognitive thought process of worry, but it is accompanied by emotional and/or physical responses too. Emotions tied to normal anxiety include fear, doubt, dread, unease, and nervousness. Physical symptoms include elevated heart rate and rapid breathing, chest tightness or palpitations, sweating, muscle tension, trembling, dizziness or lightheadedness, a sensation of butterflies in the stomach, and nausea. These symptoms are closely tied to our biological stress response and the fight-or-flight mechanism (which I'll explain below).

Often anxiety can be helpful, providing social and performance benefits. It can serve to alert us to threats and increase our vigilance in the face of potential danger or encourage us to find a solution or take action. Driving on icy roads can produce anxiety, which can lead us to focus more, drive more slowly, and be more aware of other cars and pedestrians—even as our heart pounds and breathing quickens. When a school deadline is approaching or soccer playoffs are looming, your teen may well feel anxiety in the form of worry accompanied by butterflies in their stomach, which can then motivate them to act proactively—to plan study sessions or work on practice drills. Without anxiety, they may let deadlines or practice slide and become less effective. Normal anxiety is usually short-lived, ebbing and flowing as stressors in life come and go.

The Biological Stress Response

I find that a grasp of what goes on in our bodies when we sense danger or a stressor can be helpful in understanding anxiety. In the face of threat, our body (or more precisely our autonomic nervous system) activates its biological stress response to protect us with a series of involuntary adaptive reactions, mobilizing bodily resources to confront or escape the perceived danger. The sympathetic nervous system (part of the autonomic nervous system) has two primary mechanisms—directly stimulating organs such as the heart and lungs, and triggering the release of stress hormones like adrenaline and cortisol. Together, they set off a cascade of changes across a broad range of organ systems, leading to enhanced oxygen intake, expanded lungs, increased blood flow to the muscles and brain, and greater cognitive attention and focus, which all work together to give us the best chance of survival.

Our fight-or-flight system is designed to activate in the face of danger and, when the threat has passed, to downshift to a more relaxed state. Originally, it would have been called on rarely or occasionally; there were only so many times your ancestors would run across a bear or a mammoth, or your neighbors would show up with bloody intent on their minds. But in today's world, your teen's stress response might be activated by all kinds of perceived dangers: an upcoming SAT test or a precalculus exam score. Once the test is over or the results are received, ideally their nervous system will settle down again. This was Emma's experience in lower through middle school: She experienced intense stress activation before school started and in the buildup to anxiety-inducing events, before calming down in the wake of them, until things worsened dramatically for her in high school.

Healthy stress: Stress, like anxiety, is often considered a bad thing. But some stress in life is good, even necessary. Some refer to this as *healthy stress* (or *eustress*), given that a low level of stress keeps you interested and engaged. You might experience it when starting a new job, or trying an activity for the first time, or traveling. It wards off boredom, lassitude, and laziness and contributes to personal growth. Healthy stress is not always completely comfortable, but it shouldn't cause significant *dis*tress. Stress exists along a continuum, from no stress, to healthy stress, to problematic or toxic stress.

Toxic stress: For many people, a serious problem arises when our body's stress response is activated frequently, chronically, and without relief by repeated stressors in the environment—such as a challenging relationship or job. Many of our kids face this almost every day in the cauldron of excessive school demands and achievement pressure. When the body's fight-or-flight mechanism is activated in a persistent and/or extremely intense manner, without any opportunity for rest or recovery, problems ensue. Potential effects of long-term stress include behavioral and mental health issues, such as anxiety—as in Emma's case. Toxic stress can contribute to emotional outbursts, mood swings, persistent and intrusive worry, feelings of sadness, chronic difficulties with focusing, distractibility, drug and alcohol use, risk-taking behaviors, social withdrawal, depression, PTSD, pessimism, cynicism, decrease in motivation, and sensitivity to criticism. It can also have a profound negative impact on overall health and has been linked to increased risks of high blood pressure, heart disease, diabetes, obesity, immune system suppression, digestive problems, and autoimmune conditions.[9]

When carrying out my research in schools, I was interested in exploring stress in the lives of students. I didn't want to add a specific stress instrument to the survey because it would add unnecessary length, but the anxiety scale we were using, the State portion of the State-Trait Anxiety Inventory (STAI),[10] has been found to be strongly correlated with stress. In the Silicon Valley school district that I surveyed, administrators were interested in examining this proxy measure of stress. We found that the mean score on this instrument was 46.6 in their school district (it was 50.3 in the Northern California school I first surveyed and 52.4 in the Catholic girls school). But what did these numbers mean? We turned to the original STAI manual and found the following scores: Working adults had a mean score of 35.5, college students had a 37.6, and navy recruits in their first week of basic training had a 45.5. Imagine that! Except for vacation breaks, students in these high schools were experiencing the same (or greater) level of stress *over four years* as recruits in a military basic training program. No wonder they were testing so high for anxiety and depression.

For Emma, and millions of teens like her, the relentless pressure of grind culture in high school kept her stress response system constantly activated until she was living in survival mode twenty-four hours a day. In Emma's case, her stress about starting school in tenth grade never settled down as it had in previous years, and she became anxious all the time, her young body beset by nervous tics. That unremitting stress and repeated activation of the fight-or-flight response likely led to the development of the problematic form of anxiety, known as clinical anxiety or anxiety disorders.

Clinical Anxiety and Anxiety Disorders

In some ways, the terms *clinical anxiety* and *anxiety disorders* can be used interchangeably, as they both mean that anxiety has moved beyond what might be considered normal and is significantly affecting someone's functioning in a negative way. However, I have some trouble with the term *anxiety disorder,* as it centers the problem on the person, the implication being that the disorder resides solely within them rather than, as happens in many cases, the environment they are living in. I prefer the term *clinical anxiety* because it means that anxiety has reached a stage that requires attention and treatment. That said, the *DSM-5* refers to anxiety disorders, so I'll use the term when describing them here and *clinical anxiety* elsewhere.

Generalized anxiety disorder (GAD) is the most common anxiety disorder. The thoughts, feelings, and physical symptoms associated with GAD are essentially the same as those of normal anxiety, but they are elevated in frequency and severity. For frequency, the *DSM-5* defines the cutoff as excessive anxiety and worry about events and activities that occur more days than not for at least six months. Other criteria for making the diagnosis include the presence over a six-month period of three or more physical or cognitive symptoms (only one or more symptoms required for children), such as difficulty in concentrating, restlessness, muscle tension, and sleep disturbance. GAD has two other key components—that someone has difficulty in controlling their worry (even if they know the worry is excessive) and that the anxiety, worry, and/or physical symptoms lead to significant distress or impairment in daily life.

Another important note to make here in support of using the term *clinical anxiety* is that a diagnosis of GAD requires anxiety to be present for at least six months. Technically, Emma would not have qualified because she had had symptoms for only two to three months, yet she clearly had a clinically significant degree of anxiety, and treatment was undoubtedly warranted.

Many people dismiss anxiety as inevitable, especially for teens, but it can create disruptions in multiple areas of someone's life, such as personal relationships, work, and school, and can cause substantial emotional pain. It can also contribute to a whole host of physical health problems, including cardiovascular maladies; gastrointestinal problems; chronic pain and muscle tension; sleep disturbances; weakened immune function; and increased risk for alcohol, nicotine, or other drug use/abuse. With this litany of social, emotional, and physical health problems, it goes without saying that the potential threat to one's well-being and overall satisfaction with life is large and should not be ignored.

What Can a Parent Do?

In the increasingly frenzied and pressured lives of parents and kids, it can be difficult to slow down and consider whether your child has a problem that needs professional attention. However, given the prevalence of anxiety in teens, it is a critically important step to take as a family. If you think your child is being affected by anxiety in some way, the first step is to try to determine whether it is worry, normal anxiety, or clinical anxiety.

For Worry

Worry is a purely cognitive process; and if your child is experiencing worry, they will not exhibit any physical or emotional symptoms. For many teens, worry tends to center on performance concerns in academics, sports, other extracurricular activities, and social situations. As a parent you may be aware that your child is worried because of what they say as they speak their thoughts out loud. Typical worry statements may or may not include the word *worry.* For example, a child may say, "I'm worried I'm going to fail my math test tomorrow" or "I know I'm going to fail my math exam tomorrow." However, not all kids express their worry verbally and instead may engage in actions like procrastination or overstudying, or may exhibit excess irritability.

Looking back, I have to admit that I didn't do a very good job of helping my kids with worry. If they were concerned about an exam or a sports event, I tended to use my go-to reassurance: *Don't worry, you'll do fine, you always do fine.* As my now-grown daughters would definitely agree, this approach is not effective and, moreover, can make things worse by making your child feel that you are dismissing their concerns. Instead, I recommend that you try these simple steps:

- **Validate their thoughts.** If your child is worried about a project or an upcoming exam, telling them not to worry won't take the worries away. Instead, you could say something like "That's understandable because this test feels important, and I know how challenging the material has been for you."
- **Empathize with your child.** If you see evidence of distress, try to make sure that your child understands that you recognize this. "I know this feels like a big deal, and that must be hard."
- **Probe for understanding and explore perceived negative outcomes.** Sometimes your child can get stuck in a cycle of worry without considering why exactly they are worrying—and whether it is necessary. You can get your child to consider

the root of their concern by asking, "What's the outcome you are worried about?" If they are worried about not getting an A plus on a test, you can help them explore what's driving their thoughts and whether they are realistic. Sometimes perspective checking can be useful and can rein in worries. Finding out what's driving the worry can be illuminating for you and your teen.

- **Problem-solve with them, not for them.** Our tendency as parents is to jump in to try to solve problems for our kids, giving them advice rather than supporting them in coming up with solutions themselves. Instead of leaping to potential fixes, you can ask questions such as "You're worried about your finals. Do you think it would help to feel more prepared and, if so, what could you do now?" or "Do you think taking a break might be helpful?" You can also ask, "Can I help in any way?"
- **Offer reassurance or encouragement:** Reassure and encourage them with statements like "You've got this!" or "Do the best you can!" (along with a hug if they'll tolerate it).
- **Change the subject.** Once you've validated, empathized, and encouraged, you don't have to dwell on the test or worry-provoking subject. It can be helpful for your teen to see that their concern doesn't have to take up all the oxygen in the room. There's only so much worrying that needs to be done, and turning their mind to something else can be beneficial—to everyone.

For Normal Anxiety

Normal anxiety is worry accompanied by physical and/or emotional symptoms that are short-lived and not frequent or particularly distressing, such as a trembly feeling or crying. It usually occurs in the context of high-pressure activities such as exams or sports events, or on opening night for a play or concert, or before social events. Common symptoms are nausea, headache, shakiness, or light-headedness that tend to be relatively fleeting. Typical emotional reactions include feelings of fear and tearfulness, and entreaties to avoid participation in the event if that is the source of stress. Noah, a talented high-school athlete, frequently feels nauseous before track meets and thinks up ways he can avoid competitions. His anxiety dies down as soon as he begins his races, then revs up before the next meet.

Helping kids manage normal anxiety is much the same as helping them manage worry, while paying more attention to physical and emotional symptoms that might feel distressing to them. Begin by validating, empathizing, and probing for understanding. The following approaches can be beneficial too:

- **Normalize their anxiety.** Let them know that their anxiety is understandable and that sometimes emotional and physical symptoms can accompany their worried thoughts.
- **It's their body at work.** Tell them about what's going on in their body so that if their heart is racing or they are short of breath, they can feel reassured that it's their fight-or-flight response kicking in, that it isn't dangerous and should pass quickly. This can also be an opening to demonstrate or support helpful calming techniques that can regulate their nervous system, such as the breathing exercise below.
- **Reinforce self-calming skills.**[11] There are many approaches to self-calming, several of which are widely used and evidence based, including mindfulness practice, progressive muscle relaxation, and visualization strategies. Having your teen practice staying in the present moment, rather than being distracted by worry thoughts, can help keep rumination at bay. Focusing on their breath can help your teen when they are feeling anxious. Have them try this simple, structured

deep-breathing technique known as 4-7-8 breathing. (1) breathe in for a count of four, taking a steady, deep breath; (2) hold the breath to a count of seven; (3) breathe out slowly to a count of eight; (4) repeat cycle until a calm(er) state is achieved (for me, generally four or five breath cycles).[12]

- **Encourage sleep, physical activity, and taking breaks.** Inadequate sleep can reduce resilience and can make your teen more susceptible to anxiety, so encourage bedtimes that allow for at least eight hours of sleep (or as close to eight as possible). Noncompetitive physical activity, whether walking the dog, skateboarding with friends, or engaging in low-stakes recreational sports, has also been shown to be effective at preventing and reducing anxiety in teens and is linked to enhanced cognitive functioning that can boost academic performance. Relentless study without breaks can also contribute to anxiety by causing mental fatigue and stress, so promote the idea of frequent breaks. If your child moves their body during their breaks, that's even better for their mental health—and is likely to boost their performance.

- **Be emotionally and physically present.** Make sure that your child feels like you are present in their life and available and that you have a strong sense of what they are experiencing; at the same time, avoid being intrusive or jumping too quickly to problem-solving mode. A tricky balance to master, but worth aiming for.

- **Try not to add your own anxiety to the mix.** It can be difficult to tame your own fears or concerns if your child is melting down before a big exam or track meet, but try your best to keep calm. Kids are more likely to lose control of their emotions if you do too, so aim to be a reassuring presence in the face of their anxiety episodes. You may benefit from learning deep breathing or other calming tools (I'll teach you another one in chapter 9 that I use all the time) to practice in trying situations.

For Clinical Anxiety

For some teens, normal anxiety begins to appear more frequently and to a greater degree until it seems to pervade their daily lives rather than only arising in stressful situations and then disappearing until the next time. They may be regularly anxious about going to school or participating in after-school activities, sports and other interests, or social events, and they may start to avoid situations or people that cause them distress. Over time, some behaviors can strain family relationships. These may be familiar to many of you; they include procrastination or avoidance of homework or projects, refusal to go to activities and events, withdrawal from family, or overall social withdrawal. Some kids may refuse to go to school, a phenomenon known as school refusal, which is on the rise and can cause significant disruption and conflict for families. Other signs include increased irritability and mood swings with outbursts and tantrums, as well as overreliance on parents for support and in decision-making, interfering with progress toward independence and self-sufficiency. Physical symptoms such as gastrointestinal issues or sleep disturbances may become more extreme and may get in the way of their daily life.

To some extent, anxiety has been normalized in our society, where everyone is "stressed out," especially teens in high-pressure academic environments. It may be difficult for parents to tell when normal anxiety has become clinical anxiety, but it's crucial to know that feeling anxious all or much of the time shouldn't be the norm. If you are concerned in any way about your child's anxiety, then the best approach is to seek an evaluation by a mental health professional who can recommend treatment. You could get a referral from their pediatrician, a family doctor, or their school nurse or counselor. The median age of onset for anxiety disorders in children is eleven years of age, yet treatment typically doesn't begin until the mid-to-late teenage years, so delay in seeking mental health care is common. It is widely accepted that the earlier one seeks care, the better the outcome, so I would suggest that if you're unsure, make an appointment. Even if you think your child's symptoms fall into the category of normal anxiety, therapists can be helpful in teaching techniques to keep it from progressing.

In most cases, when a child is diagnosed with clinical anxiety, some form of talk therapy is typically considered the first-line treatment. The three most commonly used forms of talk therapy, which I introduced in the last chapter, are CBT (cognitive behavioral therapy), ACT (acceptance and commitment therapy), and DBT (dialectical behavior therapy). CBT is the oldest of the three, and in many ways ACT and DBT are descendants, sometimes referred to as "third-wave" cognitive behavioral therapies. Each is different, and one or another may be a better fit based on your teenager's personality and temperament, as well as their unique challenges with anxiety. A therapist can help guide you toward the best treatment for your child, but below is a brief description of each therapy:

- **Cognitive behavioral therapy:** CBT was developed in the 1970s, and because of its longevity, it has the most robust evidence for efficacy for both anxiety and depression.[13] It is considered the gold standard treatment for both conditions by numerous medical and psychological associations, including the American Psychological Association and the American Academy for Child and Adolescent Psychiatry.[14] CBT is based on the work of Aaron Beck, a pioneering American psychiatrist, who observed in his patients that distorted thoughts and beliefs could affect feelings and behavior and contribute to depression and anxiety. The therapy he pioneered is designed to help people recognize their cognitive distortions and counter them, creating more accurate, less painful narratives. CBT typically involves weekly forty-five-minute to one-hour sessions, and a full course of treatment generally runs from twelve to twenty weeks in length, although it can vary for each person. This course can be followed by booster sessions as needed.

- **Acceptance and commitment therapy:** ACT emerged in the 1990s, saw a surge in research in the 2000s, and became a widely accepted and supported treatment for depression and anxiety in the 2010s. The evidence to support its efficacy is not as strong as that for CBT (particularly for teens), but overall, it is positive and continues to grow.[15] Like CBT, ACT involves identifying distorted thoughts and negative emotions, but rather than challenge or battle them, it teaches acceptance of them along with "cognitive defusion" which means learning to see your thoughts as just that, "thoughts." It also focuses on being mindful and engaging with the present moment, showing self-compassion, and choosing actions aligned with the person's own values. Treatment sessions are generally weekly and the course is typically shorter than CBT, lasting eight to sixteen weeks, though it can be extended for complex or chronic cases and, like CBT, can be followed by additional booster sessions. Teens who may be a good fit for ACT include those who have an interest in or openness to mindfulness practices and who are attracted to the idea of exploring values and finding meaning.

- **Dialectical behavior therapy:** DBT was developed in the late 1980s by Marsha M. Linehan, a psychologist, professor, and author, who published her first clinical trial on DBT in 1992.[16] This study involved a group of women with borderline personality disorder (BPD)—a mental health condition in which people find it difficult to regulate emotions—who were prone to self-harm and chronic suicidality. Since then, it has become widely accepted as the most effective treatment for BPD, including for teens, and in more recent years it has been adopted as a treatment of depression and anxiety in teens in some situations. DBT tends to be more time intensive and therefore more expensive than CBT or ACT and involves both individual therapy and group skills training in the following modules: (1) *mindfulness,* (2) *distress tolerance,* (3) *emotional regulation,* and (4) *interpersonal effectiveness and relationship skills.* A typical full course runs six to twelve months and includes individual therapy for one hour per week as well as two (or more) hours of group skills training per week (often with parents). Given its more intensive nature, DBT is generally not recommended over CBT or ACT for most teens, but for some teens with depression or anxiety it could be a good fit.

- **Medication:** In general, talk therapy is the first recommendation for treatment, but medications can also play a role in the management of anxiety. Selective serotonin reuptake inhibitors (SSRIs) such as fluoxetine (Prozac) or sertraline (Zoloft) are most commonly prescribed when a teen has concurrent depression, when anxiety symptoms are severe, if frequent panic attacks and/or severe insomnia occur, if talk therapy hasn't proven effective, or in the case of suicidality.[17] Sometimes kids are prescribed antianxiety medications without talk therapy. While these can be helpful in addressing anxiety in the moment, talk therapy is recommended as it can address maladaptive behaviors and mindsets that arise in conjunction with anxiety, thus managing the underlying condition.

Getting your child the professional help they need is essential if they have clinical anxiety, and you can help by reinforcing the new skills that your child is learning in therapy. You also have a vital role to play, in many ways serving as a mental health or psychological first responder. When your child is showing signs of anxiety, you can implement the same techniques outlined for worry and normal anxiety: Validate their thoughts, empathize with them, probe for understanding, and only then help with problem-solving. This approach is consistent with guidelines from Psychological First Aid, an evidence-based action plan for providing psychosocial support in the aftermath of disasters, crises, and traumatic events.[18]

Avoiding the Anxiety Dependency Trap

As many of us know, it's easy for parents to fall into a pattern of stepping in to fix things when your kid is struggling with a challenge—and we are particularly prone to doing so when anxiety is involved. Rather than teaching kids to practice self-calming techniques, we step in as calmer-in-chief, jumping to soothe and support with reassuring words and touch. And rather than encouraging them to think about how they might solve their problem, we leap in too quickly to offer *our* solutions. For example, if a teen is falling apart because they are struggling to write the first paragraph of an essay for a college application, many parents tend to plunge in to tell them what they would do rather than work with the teen to get them to solve the problem. In the short term this can prove effective, as the problem is fixed and the anxiety melts away, but in the long term it can lead to an unhealthy dependency in young adulthood that can make the process of adulting even more difficult. Many of the parents I talk to whose kids are well into adulthood tell me that their kids continue to call them when the merest "crisis" strikes—a practice these parents wouldn't have dreamed of when they themselves were young adults. I don't blame the kids, who are products of the environment we created for them. In our eagerness to help, and perhaps, to model effective problem-solving, we unwittingly created an expectation that this was our role—permanently.

If you recognize anxiety dependency in your relationship with your child, it is never too late to address it by encouraging self-calming techniques and, over time, stepping back from your role in problem-solving. You can move from calmer- and problem-fixer-in-chief to chief sideline supporter.

Addressing the Root Causes

It's important that we take advantage of the many options for treating anxiety in our kids and strive to incorporate effective parenting techniques in our daily lives, as well as longer-range strategies for family life. These alone, however, are not adequate in addressing the teen mental health crisis. For this, we need to attend to root causes: achievement culture, the excessive demands and unrelenting pressures of school and extracurricular activities, and the parts that we play as parents caught up in the grind of trying to ensure our child's success in a competitive world. It's time to acknowledge that unless we make changes to the environments that our kids are immersed in, a growing number of teens' and young adults' mental health will be threatened, their nervous systems constantly activated by overwhelming toxic stress.

When Emma's parents, after being rebuffed by the school, witnessed their daughter's pain, their response was to get her professional help to treat her anxiety—which helped. And yet they continued to keep her in a system that was hurting her because they—and she—had bought into the notion that the benefits the school could provide—prestige as an academic magnet and the accompanying rigor—could help assure her future success. In pointing this out, I don't mean to cast blame on Emma's parents—it's a dynamic that many of us operate in. Only when we assess our role as parents and call out the problems inherent in schools will things start to shift. We don't need to accept sky-high anxiety rates in kids as normal. It is well within the capacity of schools to address the high-demand, high-pressure environments and make changes that benefit students' well-being; moreover, it should be their mandate to do so! We'll explore what that looks like—and what you can take onboard in your own lives—in the coming chapters.

Part 2

A Case Study

Chapter 4

My Initiative to Combat Depression, Anxiety, and Toxic Stress in My Students

It can feel overwhelming to know how widespread the teen mental health crisis is and that it's on the rise; to see how young people are struggling; and to wonder if there's any way out of the traps they are caught in. What I have learned, though, is that solutions do exist, transformative options that are neither radical nor costly to implement, and that can make a huge difference in students' lives. At Saint Louis University School of Medicine (SLU) we were able to accomplish tangible changes that brought about enormous improvements in our students' well-being. In the pages that follow I'll tell you how we made it happen. The lessons learned from that experience are directly relevant to addressing teens' and preteens' distress, for the issues they face are similar.

One afternoon in 2008, I pulled a chair over and sat down next to my colleague and friend John Chibnall. It was near the end of the academic year, and Chibnall was about to share the results of the mental health screening survey we had recently administered to our students. I had arrived at SLU four years earlier as associate dean for curriculum and, as part of my role, had become well versed in medical education research articles reporting high rates of depression, anxiety, burnout, and suicidal ideation in U.S. medical students. The numbers were dismal. Studies found that 49.6 percent met criteria for burnout, 25 to 33 percent were anxious, 13 to 25 percent were depressed, and 11.2 percent reported suicidal ideation, meaning that they had had thoughts of taking their own life in the past year.[1] I wasn't concerned that we had such high rates at *our* school. I knew the students at SLU. There were some who struggled with their mental health, but the vast majority seemed to be happy, even thriving. They smiled when passing me in the halls and chatted with me between classes. I had worked hard to create a supportive environment in which students felt respected, heard, and cared for, and we had an excellent counseling center if treatment was needed. Our baseline surveys of our first-year students, taken during orientation week at the start of the academic year, indicated that student mental health overall had looked fairly good, with a depression rate of only 6 percent. The anxiety rate of 33 percent was markedly higher but not surprising, as the students all knew they were about to enter an intense, challenging, and demanding year. In the face of that, having a degree of anxiety was, in some ways, a reasonable reaction.

Chibnall clicked through several open windows on his desktop screen and pulled up the document with the end-of-year survey results. I scanned the table to find the numbers. First-year students, depression rate 27 percent; second-years, 29 percent. And for anxiety, first-years, 56 percent; second-years, 58 percent. I slumped back in my chair, astounded. Our students were not doing well at all.

Then it hit me: Not only were they struggling, but *we were doing this to them.* We had created an environment that had caused their mental health to plummet and then stay that way. The first-years' scores had increased drastically since they'd arrived at SLU just nine months earlier, with depression rates more than quadrupling. As curriculum dean, I grasped that I was ultimately responsible. I knew wholeheartedly that I could not be in charge of an educational enterprise that produced such poor mental health outcomes in our students. Our mission statement was to educate the whole person—mind, body, spirit, and heart—and clearly we were failing. Worse, we were hurting our students. I knew things had to change.

For the next six years I devoted my time and attention to transforming those outcomes, understanding what was contributing to our students' high rates of depression and anxiety, and learning what we could do as a school to improve their well-being. The lessons we learned, the nature of the changes we implemented, and the theory behind them, as well as the politics involved, are vital to consider for the current youth mental health crisis.

Reducing Stress

Our year-end survey of students was a wake-up call, but it also provided us some potential paths forward. In addition to questions about depression and anxiety symptoms, we'd asked the students to rate the level of stress caused by a variety of factors. The three stressors that rose to the top were, in rank order:

1. The volume of information in their courses
2. The level of detail of the material
3. Competition for grades

These were not surprising results. In the U.S., the first two years of medical school focus intensely on the basic sciences (biochemistry, anatomy, physiology) and the clinical sciences (pathology, pathophysiology, pharmacology), and the diagnosis and management of hundreds upon hundreds of diseases. An inordinate amount of information was unleashed on the students, and learning it was, in many ways, akin to trying to memorize huge quantities of new material in an unfamiliar language.

The level of detail that (some) faculty expected the students to grasp was extraordinary—and unrealistic. They would teach for two hours on subjects that they had studied for years, and they expected the students to have a comparable level of understanding, even while knowing there was a whole lineup of other faculty demanding the same for their own area of expertise. Engaging this curriculum with the intent and expectation of mastering it has been described as drinking from a fire hose. When you add to it the exponential increase of scientific knowledge in the past half century, the situation starts to resemble an absurdity—or worse, a form of torture such as waterboarding, as a physician assistant student at SLU described it.

The third-highest-ranked stressor for our medical students was competition for grades. We had a four-tier grading system that included Honors, High Pass, Pass, and Fail designations. Most medical schools at the time employed a variation of this grading system, though some had three tiers and others had five. It was intended to motivate student performance, allowing students to strive for one of the higher tiers—but it also had a downside. In many ways, medical students represent the pinnacle of achievement culture, having been extremely successful in their academic studies in high school and college, motivated to be diligent and dedicated students to get into medical school, and still driven on arrival. Competition among these high-flying students could be fierce, contributing to extra stress and leading some to feel average or below average for the first time in their lives. As we'll explore in the next chapter, not meeting one's own expectations and standards can contribute to significant distress and lead to obsessive studying habits where sleep and personal health are compromised.

With a clear understanding of what was stressing out our students, I started to look for potential remedies for their mental health problems. Like a good academician, I jumped into the medical education literature. My search took me back to the 1930s. Soon a history of different attitudes and approaches comprising three main phases became evident to me. The first phase stretched from the 1930s into the 1960s, and the prevailing attitude was that life is tough; medicine is tough; so, if you're struggling with your mental health, suck it up or get out of the field. In the next phase there was a recognized need to provide mental health services to medical students and to promote their access and utilization. Medical schools across the country (including SLU) ramped up their psychological services—a significant step forward. The third phase began, roughly speaking, in the 2000s, and included changes to pass/fail grading systems in a few places and the institution and development of "wellness" programs. These programs have since grown dramatically over the years and are now ubiquitous in medical schools nationally. They were designed to help students live healthier lives using strategies that emphasize physical health—good nutrition, exercise, and sleep practices, regular visits to primary care doctors and dentists—and mental health maintenance using approaches such as mindfulness.

To a substantial degree, we had these robust mental health and wellness interventions in place already at SLU. Our students had excellent access to mental health services. Our kind and beloved assistant dean of student affairs, Jim Swierkosz, organized and enthusiastically participated in activities meant to foster high morale among the students, including social gatherings and impromptu events, such as mini-golf in the hallways of our learning resource center. His colleague Greg Smith, a surgically trained scientist, teacher, course director, and mentor, was always available to students and had their backs. We had tried hard to create an environment where students could let off steam and get help and treatment when they needed it. However, it was clear that these well-intentioned efforts were not sufficient to protect their mental health and well-being in the face of the stress of the intensive medical school curriculum we subjected them to and the relentless pressure brought on by peer competition.

Across the country today, countless high schools follow this same approach—encouraging the use of mental health treatment for students with anxiety and depression and providing social support to try to prop them up when they flag. It was clear to me then as it is now that treating mental health issues in the aftermath of extreme stress is not enough, whether in high school, college, or graduate school. We needed to get ahead of the problem and address the educational environment. A new model was required.

Changing the Environment

If we wanted to make a difference in our students' well-being, we needed to listen to what they were telling us—and act upon it.

First, we had to address the onerous course load. But how? It is widely acknowledged in medical education circles that cutting content is a third-rail proposition, meaning it's untouchable, something that one undertakes at one's peril. It is an unpopular solution, for it can easily represent an affront to a medical faculty's strongly held views of what is essential to a functional knowledge of their field and their belief that any cut in content would be a lowering of standards. The modus operandi has always been the more, the better, both in volume and in detail, which has its roots in an understanding—or, more accurately, a misunderstanding—that requiring mastery of an excessive amount of information leads to better outcomes, and therefore that requiring less leads to worse outcomes. This premise is false, as I'll describe later in the chapter, and yet it has had remarkable staying power, contributing significantly to a bias toward overload in curricula of medical schools, colleges, universities, and, of course, the portal that leads to them all—high schools. This attachment to excessive content is prevalent in high schools where some teachers might teach from college textbooks or where students are pressured to take as many AP courses as possible and therefore overload their schedules in order to stand out. For high school students, the rule seems to be that if one hour of homework is good, then two hours must be better, and four hours must be better still. The research on homework proves otherwise, as I'll describe in chapter 8.

I was confident that we could reduce content at SLU (both the volume and the level of detail) without harming our educational outcomes—which is to say, not lowering standards. In fact, if I was correct in believing that we were overloading our students unnecessarily, then unloading unnecessary content should not decrease learning; it might even enhance it!

Our next issue was the question of competition for grades. During my research, I had taken note of a growing trend in medical education toward a pass/fail grading system for the first- and second-years and wondered if it might work for us. Some 40 percent of medical schools had already implemented this system. Among the early adopters, the University of Virginia, Mayo Medical School, and the University of Michigan had evaluated its effects, and all three had come up with the same finding: There was no drop in academic performance at all as measured by scores on internal exams as well as on the National Board of Medical Examiners Step 1 exam at the end of the first two years of medical school.[2] While their studies did not assess depression or anxiety in response to the change, student satisfaction, well-being, or stress levels had improved in each case. That was exactly what we were looking for.

Given the backbone of evidence, both demonstrated and theoretical, which supported that reducing content and eliminating grades would not harm student performance and, moreover, could reduce stress, I felt as if we had a sound basis for moving forward with proposing a plan. If we could decrease the amount of material and the level of detail that students were expected to learn and move to a pass/fail grading system, we would change the toxic environment that was affecting students so negatively. In doing so, I was hopeful that we would make significant strides toward improving student mental health.

However, I was also aware that changing the learning environment wouldn't be enough. Medical school would still be demanding, and the students' future residency training would be stressful as they gained hands-on experience with patients in all kinds of medical situations, as would their future medical practice. It wouldn't make sense for us to focus solely on reducing stress in one environment, knowing that they would be exposed to new stressors for the rest of their professional (and personal) lives. Our goal would be to lower and ideally eliminate unnecessary and toxic stress but not to make the experience stress-free. We needed to try to provide students with the ability to better *handle* stress. An approach that I felt had potential was to teach our students cognitive restructuring, the core technique used by therapists in cognitive behavioral therapy, and a first-line treatment of anxiety and depression. We didn't have enough therapists to provide individual care to the entire student body, and the reality was that some students wouldn't seek treatment even if they needed it, because of perceived stigma or other reasons. We decided then to see if we could teach *all* the students these techniques and potentially help *prevent* the onset of depression and anxiety in some.

In addition, there was one piece that I felt was still missing and that I sensed intuitively was important. I believed that we needed to create opportunities for our students to find meaning in their work, to rediscover some of their initial passion for medicine. I could imagine that their lives of constant study and stress were lacking in basic joy and fulfillment. From my own experience as a physician and medical educator, I had a strong conviction that this would be protective for their mental health. I had felt fortunate to work in a profession where I had the opportunity to make a difference in other people's lives, whether kids, parents, or students, to find meaning beyond my own life, and that had helped sustain me during the long hours and challenges of my career. I was profoundly influenced by the writings of Viktor Frankl, whom I had come across years before during the stressful and demanding period that characterized my final years as a faculty member at UCLA.

Frankl was a German psychiatrist, author, philosopher, and concentration camp survivor who developed logotherapy, a form of psychotherapy grounded in helping patients find a sense of meaning in their lives. In his landmark book of 1946, *Man's Seach for Meaning,* he wrote one of my favorite quotes, one that I still use today in many of my talks: "There is nothing in the world, I venture to say, that would so effectively help one to survive even the worst conditions as the knowledge that there is a meaning in one's life. There is much wisdom in the words of Nietzsche, 'He who has a why to live for can bear almost any how.' "[3] The question—my question—became, How could we structure the students' courses and time to allow them to find that meaning, to engage in electives, community service, or research that would ignite their sense of purpose?

With this final piece, we had a three-pronged plan to pressure-proof our students, one that brought the school and the students themselves into the process: Improve the learning environment, increase students' resilience, and bring meaning and joy to their lives.

The Interventions

One academic year later, we were ready to implement our changes. We had decided to begin with the learning environment, bringing on board four integrated (and hopefully synergistic) modifications, starting with our first-year students:

- An across-the-board 10 percent cut in class time during the first two curricular years, which would free up every other Wednesday for electives and personal time
- A reduction in the amount of detail taught in classes
- An adjustment to a simple pass/fail grading system
- The creation of five theme-based learning communities in areas such as research, community service, and global health, in which students and faculty with common interests could work together in elective courses, hold noon seminars and talks, and collaborate on projects

We planned to add our resilience curriculum to the mix a year later for the incoming first-year class so we could measure our results more effectively. It would consist of a presentation on maladaptive mindsets, cognitive distortions, and managing thoughts and emotions; a talk on mindfulness techniques; and some time dedicated to small group work.

The Obstacles

Getting to the implementation stage in such a short time was nothing short of a miracle, but we felt that the mission was urgent, and knowing how our students were struggling lit a fire beneath our feet. That said, it was not an easy journey—effecting change never is—and we seemed to meet resistance at every turn.

Tradition

The decision to move forward with our sweeping set of changes had not rested solely in my hands. I needed approval from three committees—the Curriculum Management, Curriculum Oversight, and Executive Committees of the Medical School—and the last of these was notoriously traditionalist in its bent. The culture within medical education has been characterized by a long history of glacially paced curricular change. At its core has been the well-intentioned principle to uphold the highest standards of excellence, whatever the cost, and adding and maintaining course content and performance pressure has been erroneously—and understandably—seen as a key to this. Knowing that there would be resistance to my proposed changes, I included a fail-safe with my plan that I believed could make it more acceptable to the faculty and the governing committees: If, in two years, we found that student academic performance had dropped, we would add back the curricular time and content and revert back to the old grading system.

Entrenched Ideas

The students themselves had to be won over when it came to moving to pass/fail. We had to address their fears that doing away with grades would make them less competitive for residency programs, as well as their concern that excellence wouldn't be rewarded, that they would lose their drive without external motivators, or that dispensing with grades could be un-American somehow, an approach that could make students lazy and soft. Their resistance made sense. After all, grades had been a part of their lives since childhood, and the vast majority had gotten not only good grades but *great* grades, almost perfect grades, their entire lives. They were the best and the brightest, the academic elite who had triumphed in the scholastic races in high school, college, and even earlier, in middle and elementary school. They were the "smart ones," to whom parents had pointed with open pride throughout their childhood, often to the chagrin of their less academically talented siblings. For (too) many of them, grades weren't evidence of their achievement; they were an integral part of their *identity*. It was therefore no surprise that some students were reluctant to give up grades. Without these guideposts, these tokens of validation in the eyes of society and themselves, who and what would they be?

But the truth was that grades had predictable adverse effects, encouraging toxic competition among the students (which had caused so many of them stress in the first place) and even straining relationships with faculty, who often had to strenuously defend anything less than an honors grade. Also, with grades, there was no end point; you could always learn more, memorize more, to try to achieve that honors grade that was conferred on the top 20 percent of the class. With pass/fail grading in place, we could hope to counteract that.

Change Takes Effort

There was an enormous amount of work involved in planning, reflecting, educating the various parties, considering competing points of view, completing research, and choosing the best path. Over the course of the year, many people threw their hearts and souls into trying to do what we felt was right. We carried out a student survey on the grading system, held a student town hall, initiated multiple faculty forums, and presented research findings at several committee meetings.

In the end, I was able to sway the three committees to adopt our proposed changes in unanimous positive votes.

The Results at One Year

At the end of the first year, I was glad to report that all the changes related to the learning environment were implemented for our first-year students: pass/fail grading; 10 percent cut in the curriculum; every other Wednesday for electives and discretionary time. Everything had gone smoothly, and we had noticed some encouraging results.

Collaboration

I had seen evidence of more collaborative work between students, who now viewed their classwork and exams as a collective challenge rather than a competition, particularly now that they weren't all trying to edge one another out of the top 20 percent. A student put together a flow chart to help fellow students understand a complicated enzymatic process. Another provided mnemonics to help with memorization of particularly obscure and difficult-to-memorize facts. As students no longer saw their classmates as competitors, cooperation like this among them soared. There was absolutely no incentive for them to compete with one another in a pass/fail system, as their scores didn't matter except as a rough guide to how much they were learning. Relationships with faculty improved also, as students spent time working with them in the learning center and there was no longer any reason to challenge faculty in an effort to gain points for a final grade.

Finding Meaning

The students embraced the new learning communities, pursuing nascent interests and following their curiosity, and a bevy of self-designed electives emerged, ranging from mentoring and tutoring elementary school kids to creating a medical student vegetable garden accompanied by the development of healthy diet recommendations.

A group of students launched a program that brought high school students into the medical school labs, where they learned to suture and tie knots—giving the teens an exciting taste of life beyond the classroom. Others started a nonprofit organization called MEDLaunch, a biomedical and entrepreneurship incubator that grew to include students in the Schools of Business, Law, and Engineering, Aviation, and Technology, creating a wonderful intersection of ideas and learning.[4] The students' medical knowledge connected them to a world beyond the classroom, one where they were making a significant impact, and their collective energy, excitement, and passion were palpable. And it wasn't only serious endeavors that students became engaged in; four second-year students formed a band called The Palpations, finding balance and joy in playing music and performing together.[5]

Autonomy

Our students had much more autonomy in their lives—in their elective opportunities where they could follow interests, but also in a newfound independence in considering how much and what to study. Rather than chasing a score, a grade, or a class ranking, they could decide when they had learned enough or when to dig deeper into a topic. In addition, we had noticed that they were experiencing new ways of feeling competent about themselves in their elective activities, rather than relying on test scores and grades to define themselves. They had pushed themselves in different directions, developed new strengths, and grown as humans.

But the big question remained: Would the changes translate into improved mental health for our students as we hoped? Only the numbers would show. At the end of the year, we had administered our mental health survey as usual, and, with the results in, it was time for the proverbial moment of truth. Had our modifications made a dent in the depression and anxiety rates?

Mental Health Outcomes

As Chibnall pulled up the report on his computer in his cramped office, I stood over his shoulder to watch, holding my breath. We had made the changes for the first-year class but not for the second-years, so an improvement in mental health compared to the previous year's numbers for the first-years could indicate if they had been effective. First-year student depression rates: 19 percent, down from an average of 27 percent from the previous two years. And anxiety rates were 44 percent, down from 55 percent. I breathed out. Not bad. And second-year rates? They remained poor with no improvement, as expected. It was clear that our efforts had paid off; we were on the right track. But there remained much more work to be done, for while the results indicated a clear improvement, the numbers and the suffering that lay behind them were still too great.

Adding the Resilience Program

The following year, we introduced our resilience curriculum to the new first-year class while keeping the previous changes to course material and grading in effect for both first- and second-years. The cognition presentation on problematic mindsets and cognitive distortions was well received (and I'll elaborate on it in the next two chapters), but some students voiced their displeasure with the mindfulness presentation and the small group work, saying that it was a waste of time and took away from their study time. While the full program didn't feel entirely successful, I was hopeful that it might have reached and even helped some of the students. When I went over to Chibnall's office at the end of the year for what was becoming an annual ritual, he pulled up the results of the latest survey on his computer screen and we dove in. First, the first-year students: They had experienced the grading system changes, a cut in class time, the new electives, *and* the resilience curriculum. The depression numbers: 18 percent—essentially the same as the 19 percent seen the year before (but down from 32 percent of two years earlier). The resilience curriculum hadn't really made a difference. But what about anxiety? The year before it had been 44 percent and this year it was 30 percent! It was down a lot from the year before, but when compared to the baseline year rates of 55 percent, it was a huge decline! The resilience curriculum, even though some students had *hated* aspects of it, seemed to have broken through and made a real difference. I sat for a second with Chibnall and savored the numbers.

My curiosity soon pushed my attention onward as I was eager to see the results for the second-years. They hadn't experienced the resilience curriculum, but they did have the other changes that had continued into their second year. As Chibnall scrolled ahead to find their numbers, we recalled that depression rates from the prior two years had averaged 31 percent. And now they were down to 17 percent, a huge drop! I was less confident that anxiety rates would decrease, as we had surveyed the students right before they started their dedicated study period for Step 1 of the boards—an eight-hour exam that would test them on their acquired medical knowledge to date, a stressor I could do nothing to change. Anxiety might be considered an appropriate anticipatory emotion to have. The results confirmed my suspicion: The anxiety rate was 61 percent, as high as the previous year.

Other Changes

We continued to make changes over the next several years, seeing what might bring down our numbers further. We made revisions to our resilience curriculum, based on student feedback, reducing the focus on mindfulness and eliminating the small group sessions. The problematic mindset and cognitive distortion topics and tools that we introduced in the first year were revisited and reinforced in presentations at key transition points during the second year and beyond: in the run-up to the Step 1 exam; during orientation week preceding the clerkship year (the third year); and just before graduation during the fourth-year required capstone course that prepares students for their first year of residency. These presentations were supplemented by occasional, brief in-class messages and "pep talks" that I gave, as well as in e-mails, which I sent to the class listservs periodically as various stressors arose.

We also addressed a toxic course—which I'll define as one in which the demands are inordinately high and/or the grading scheme is too harsh. Our human anatomy course hit the mark on both of these criteria and was causing our students undue stress. Toxic courses are not unique to medical school; my two daughters experienced at least one in every semester during high school. The reasons vary—a teacher might require that students master an outrageous quantity of content, assign huge amounts of homework, and/or grade tests or exams harshly—but the results are the same: unnecessary student stress. At SLU, human anatomy was the first course of the first year for students, and for many it served as a rough introduction to medical school. I didn't have the power to get the course directors to change, but my boss, the dean of the medical school, did. He told them in no uncertain terms to ease the pressure and make the exams less difficult. I'm happy to report that the course directors complied, and human anatomy changed from an extremely toxic course to a moderately toxic one, which, when combined with moving it from the first course of the year to the second, dramatically decreased stress on students.

Our Results Five Years On

Mental Health

Five years in, the first-year students' depression rate had dropped from 27 percent to 4 percent, and the second-year students' from 32 percent to 6 percent.[6] Anxiety rates for first-years had decreased from 55 percent to 14 percent, and second-years' from 60 percent to 31 percent—the latter figure somewhat elevated but understandably so, as the students had taken the survey right before they entered their study period for the first installment of the national board exam. Behind these astonishing numbers were stories of real lives transformed. One first-year student told me that she had suffered with anxiety and depression throughout her high school and college years and that at SLU her mental health problems had been greatly alleviated. When she had gone home for Thanksgiving break, her mother had told her that she felt like she had her daughter back. It was exciting and moving to hear such words.

We were also able to see how our students were doing compared to other U.S. medical students through the Association of American Medical Colleges (AAMC) annual national survey of second-year medical students.[7] The survey didn't ask about signs of depression and anxiety, but it did screen for burnout symptoms of exhaustion and disengagement, which are reasonable proxies to assess overall mental health and well-being. When the results were published our numbers looked great: Our exhaustion and disengagement levels were much lower than the national average. What was also striking was our students' assessment of how they spent their time. SLU students reported getting half an hour more of sleep per night than the average med student, and they reported spending *one and a half to two hours less per day in class or studying.*

We were delighted. Our three-pronged approach had made a huge difference in the lives of our students.

Academic Performance

The big, looming question, of course, was, What happened to our students' academic performance? Surely, with fewer class hours and less content to learn, something had to give, and most people would assume that academic standards fell. And this is perhaps the sweetest part of the story. Not only did academic performance not fall, it *improved*! Our students' mean score on the huge national board exam increased, paralleling an increase nationally, and the failure rate on the exam fell by half—to 2 percent, which was half that of the national average.

Our students also found great success in residency placements. It's difficult to quantify, but there was subjective improvement there too. Many students had meaningful elective experiences that they could write and talk about in their applications and interviews. Admissions committees love when they can see evidence of genuine student passion.

The argument for ratcheting up academic pressure and workload in terms of quantity and complexity, whether in medical school or high school, has always been that it's necessary to maintain academic excellence. It just isn't true—and we had the proof. We couldn't have been happier—it meant that we could keep our changes in place and continue to support our students' well-being while providing them with a high-quality education. The scientist in me wanted to know how it could happen. How could we teach less and have students learn more? In retrospect, the answer to the question seems obvious.

First, excessive stress, sleep deprivation, exhaustion, depression, and anxiety are not supportive of cognitive functioning and learning. Over time, exposure to stress can negatively affect the ability to focus, form or retrieve memories, think flexibly, or learn[8]—all vitally important skills for medical students. One study showed that people with high stress levels were 37 percent more likely to have poor cognition.[9] I'll look at the importance of sleep and how sleep deficits can affect academic performance in chapter 9.

In addition, there is a limit to what the human brain can effectively take on. More than one hundred years ago, psychologists Robert M. Yerkes and John Dillingham Dodson illustrated this principle in their eponymous curve. The Yerkes-Dodson law describes the relationship between stress and performance, stating that performance increases with stress, but only up to a certain point. When stress is too high, performance plummets. There has been some critique of this law in recent years regarding its oversimplification and whether its original findings in animals can transfer directly to humans, but I find it provides a helpful framework for understanding how stress affects performance. I should also state that Yerkes was prominent in the eugenics movement and that some of his scientific theories, especially on intelligence, contributed to harmful and racist ideologies of the early twentieth century.

In the graph opposite, academic performance is found on the vertical axis, and academic demands and pressure occupy the horizontal axis. As you can see when you follow the curve from left to right, initially as demands and pressure increase, performance rises as someone is motivated and focused, but then as demands and pressure continue to escalate, the rise in performance levels off and then starts to decline. As demands and pressure levels grow even more, performance levels go down, and exhaustion and, eventually, burnout set in.

We tend to believe that more is always better, that more of something will always lead to better performance, but *there are few, if any, human endeavors in which this is true.* If you add too much, performance will eventually level off and then start to drop, as does mental health alongside it. As we saw in chapter 3, some stress is good and necessary in life. The same is true for class time and homework. But clearly, twenty-three hours of class and homework per day would not lead to increased learning.

Academic Performance Curve
(adapted from Yerkes-Dodson Curve)

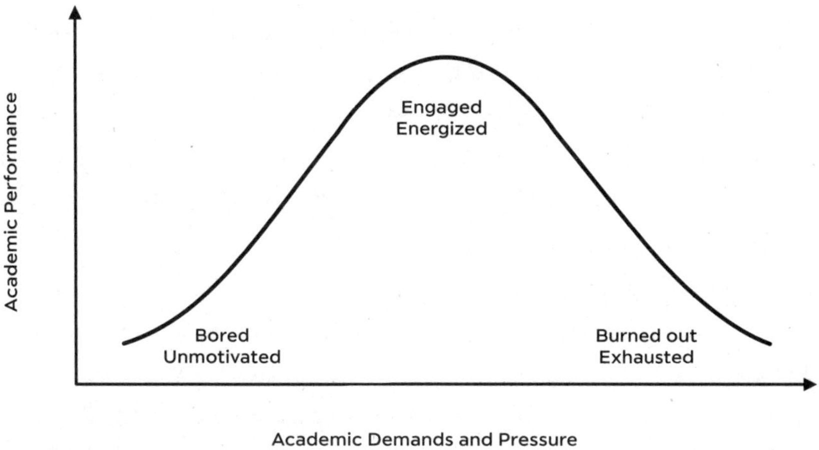

There is an upper limit—and it is likely much lower than the twelve to eighteen hours that many high schoolers put in every day as they go to school and after-school activities and then turn to homework. It can be helpful to think about the world of sports as a comparison. Of course, athletes want to work hard to build endurance, expertise, and strength, to get their reps in, but every good trainer knows the importance of rest and recovery days. They also know that at some point, after too many hours of practice or performances, the body stops working effectively and is vulnerable to breakdown and injury.

Far too few education systems are willing to try to find the sweet spot for class time, homework, and extracurriculars, one that encourages growth while facilitating well-being. Many prefer instead to continue with "more is better" and are willing to accept those who struggle or drop out as collateral damage. At SLU, as in the majority of medical schools and countless high schools across the country, we were initially too far on the right side of the Academic Performance Curve, with our students' performance moving from engaged and energized to exhausted and burned out. Counterintuitively, as our results showed, if we pull back on the pressure, we can actually increase performance.

One more outcome at SLU that I want to share is the one I am perhaps most proud of. On the AAMC Graduation Questionnaire, given to all graduating medical students in the U.S., students are asked how much they agree with the following statement: "My medical school has done a good job of fostering and nurturing my development as a person." In my last year at SLU, 33.8 percent of students nationally strongly agreed—but at SLU an astonishing 65.0 percent did. Our changes were well established by then and were continuing to make a significant positive impact on our students' lives. In my travels across the country visiting medical centers and giving talks and workshops, it is not uncommon for me to reconnect with former students, and they routinely express enormous gratitude for their educational experience at SLU. I think that what the majority are most grateful for is the support not only for their mental health and their academic achievement but for the personal growth they experienced that continued after their graduation. That is something that schools across the educational continuum can aspire to.

In the years since I left SLU, I came to realize that the many ills in medical education that we strove to combat and reverse also affect the educational and extracurricular system for our kids. The three core principles that we used at SLU to bring down depression and anxiety rates will drive and inform the rest of this book:

- **Teach, reinforce, and support resilience skills.** Help kids recognize and better manage problematic mindsets, distorted thoughts, and narrow goal setting that can lead to and increase their distress. Even though the learning environment is contributing significantly to the teen mental health crisis, kids nonetheless need effective tools to manage their reactions to it as well as to the inevitable challenges they will continue to face in life.

- **Reduce demands and pressure.** Many schools and parents ascribe to the "more is always better" principle in terms of schoolwork and extracurricular activities, which translates into an unnecessary burden on kids. The academic and achievement pressures kids feel are enormous and unhealthy, and steps must be taken to address the entire culture that is contributing to this problem. Parents need particularly to understand the importance of reducing pressure.

- **Give kids more control and more choice, and create opportunities for them to find meaning and joy in their lives.** Currently, many teens and young adults have little to no autonomy in the overly structured lives that we have created for them. We've crowded out opportunities for kids to engage in activities that bring them joy, that could give them a sense of purpose. Meaning can help sustain people, especially during difficult times, and we need to open space for this in our kids' lives.

In the next chapters, I'll keep coming back to these three concepts as we take a closer look at the harried lives our kids experience. Crucially, I'll provide key takeaways that you can begin to use immediately to make a difference for your child—and yourself.

Part 3

Finding Solutions

Chapter 5

Problematic Mindsets: The Thought Patterns That Can Trap Kids

Katherine, a first-year medical student, came to talk to me about her academic struggles. Before our meeting, I had looked quickly at her record and seen that she appeared to be doing fine, generally near the class average with no failures or near failures. Nothing stood out for me as a red flag, and I wondered what she could be struggling with. Perhaps she was working hard and was exhausted by the effort. Or she was concerned about what would come next. It can be hard to adjust to the relentless pace of medical school. When Katherine entered my office, I noticed a somewhat pained and chagrined look on her face, not unusual for a student having a difficult time—it was often challenging for them to summon the courage to open up to someone in administration. I tried to put her at her ease, welcoming her to my office and asking what brought her in. She shrugged and grimaced a little. "I'm just really unhappy with my performance," she said, "and I don't know what to do. I'm putting in a lot of hours, but it isn't translating into improvement and I'm not sure if I can push any harder."

"But Katherine, you're doing fine!" I said. "I'm not concerned with your performance at all. Your scores are right around the mean."

"I know," she said. "And that's the problem. That just doesn't feel okay to me."

Being average was a new and uncomfortable place for Katherine, who, like most medical students, was used to being on top academically. She was twenty-six, and it was likely that since kindergarten she had been one of the smartest kids in school, someone who had excelled in class and had, at least in part, defined herself around this image. We explored the feelings she was having about what she viewed as her mediocre performance, and she confessed to feeling ashamed. "I'm just so embarrassed by myself."

I was stunned. This intelligent, capable young woman was feeling *shame* about a perfectly adequate academic performance in a well-regarded medical school in a pass/fail curriculum in which her performance would not be shared with anyone outside of the school. It was akin to making it to nationals as a college athlete and feeling shame about getting a bronze medal. How could she view herself so differently than I did?

In many ways, that incident led me to explore and try to understand problematic mindsets, how they skew our view of ourselves and the world and negatively affect our lives. They are common among medical students like Katherine, as well as college and high school students—I found that the majority of high schoolers in my surveys struggled with at least one problematic mindset. As I'll describe in this chapter, they can contribute to considerable emotional pain that can lead to or exacerbate mental illness. A number of these mindsets have been shown to have very strong associations with depression and anxiety, and they are likely contributing significantly to the mental health crisis we are seeing in our youth. It's clear to me from my conversations with young people and their parents that these problematic mindsets add to, or even multiply, the distress caused by the pressured environments so many kids now experience.

Since my meeting with Katherine, I have studied four key mindsets—maladaptive perfectionism, impostor phenomenon, performance as identity, and toxic comparison—and I'll explore each of them in the pages that follow. I have found that they often work in concert, so it's not unusual for someone to have more than one, or even all of them.

What Are Problematic Mindsets?

As I said in chapter 1, mindsets are cognitive processes that can be thought of as mental filters or mental models that shape the stories we tell ourselves about our performance, our lives, and who we are. Some are positive and are associated with well-being and resilience, such as a growth-oriented (rather than fixed) mindset, optimism, self-compassion, acceptance, and gratitude. Mindsets can also be problematic and can have a distorting effect on our self-perception and our reality, bringing about negative interpretations that can cause and intensify distress.

People are not born with particular mindsets; instead, these develop and evolve in response to the environment that we live in—shaped by our parents, families, communities, schools, and society. In the U.S., success is often defined in materialistic terms and has many of us scrambling toward perfection. The problematic mindsets that I'll address in this chapter appear to be occurring at earlier ages, with numerous parents reporting that they have seen them in kids as young as six.

A core driver of this development is our education system, which relentlessly measures, sorts, and ranks kids' academic performance through tracking and standardized testing initiated as part of the No Child Left Behind (NCLB) Act enacted in 2002. Although NCLB testing does not begin until third grade, some schools are testing kindergartners and first and second graders, following the belief that introducing the tests earlier will better prepare kids for the tests to come. In reality, all it does is teach our youngest kids that they will be tested, measured, and compared constantly—and that their performance matters a lot to many adults. Testing of various kinds continues throughout elementary and middle school, ramping up, as we know, during the high school years. Even as kids bear the brunt of this pressure in school, their parents feel similarly pressured to launch their child successfully, leading to additional stress for kids at home. In turn, kids themselves can internalize societal and parental pressure, causing it to build further. Add to this the amplifying effects of social media, where kids can feel continually compared to others in their academic, extracurricular, and social achievements, and you get a sense of the overwhelm that so many kids struggle with. In this familiar pattern of contagious stress about performance, the pressures of school and achievement are responsible not just for the direct distress they cause but also, as we'll see, for fostering and nurturing the development of mindsets that exacerbate the distress—which makes teens more susceptible to the pressured school environment itself.

Below, we explore four problematic mindsets: (1) maladaptive perfectionism; (2) impostor phenomenon; (3) performance as identity; and (4) toxic comparison.

Maladaptive Perfectionism

Maladaptive perfectionism is probably the best-studied problematic mindset, and ever since my first conversation with Katherine, my first-year medical student, it has intrigued me. There is strong evidence that it is highly prevalent, not just in the U.S., but around the globe, and is on the rise. It was frequently experienced by teens in my surveys, and it comes up a lot in conversations I have with parents and high schoolers. A meta-analysis published in 2019 found that perfectionism rose in college students in the U.S., Canada, and the U.K. between 1989 and 2016.[1] In her book *Never Enough: When Achievement Culture Becomes Toxic—and What We Can Do About It,* Jennifer Breheny Wallace describes the rise in perfectionism, especially socially prescribed perfectionism driven by intense achievement culture. Maladaptive perfectionism very likely contributes to the development of depression and anxiety, but depression and anxiety can also potentially lead to the development of this mindset, setting in play a toxic cycle that is hard to break.

As its name suggests, maladaptive perfectionism is linked to perfectionism, which can be defined as striving for excellence or for success. In many ways, perfectionism is considered a positive character trait, one that motivates us to exert ourselves to do our best work—and is applauded by parents and teachers alike. This is seen as healthy or adaptive perfectionism. However, when perfectionism becomes excessive, leading us to set bars so high that failure is all but guaranteed, and causing undue stress (such as a fear of letting oneself or others down), it is known as maladaptive perfectionism.

There are several different forms of perfectionism:

Self-oriented: This form is characterized by high internal standards and harsh self-criticism. Katherine was largely suffering from self-oriented maladaptive perfectionism, her own personal standards—and her sense of failure—driving her distress.

Socially prescribed: With this kind, someone feels that others have high expectations for them, that there is a sense of pressure to be perfect in everything they do. It is combined with a fear of failing and being judged harshly. Kids and teens can suffer from socially prescribed perfectionism that stems from parents who place excessive achievement pressures on them, but it can also come from overzealous teachers and coaches as well as from society at large. When many selective colleges seem to admit only students with perfect GPAs and test scores, as well as demonstrated perfection in their (multiple) extracurriculars, it's easy to see how teens can feel the pressure to be perfect all the time.

Other oriented: This type of perfectionism occurs when someone places unrealistic standards and expectations on others and harshly judges those who don't meet these expectations. Other-oriented perfectionism is not prevalent in teens, but it is fairly common in adults who engage with kids, whether teachers, coaches, or parents, and can contribute to the development of socially prescribed and self-oriented perfectionism in children.

I've found examples of all three kinds of perfectionism in my work and my conversations with adolescents and parents, and all are relevant in the examination of teen mental health. In this chapter, I'll focus largely on self-oriented maladaptive perfectionism as it's the one that seems to occur most frequently, but I will also touch upon the other forms in my parenting advice.

Self-Oriented Maladaptive Perfectionism

Self-oriented maladaptive perfectionism is just what it sounds like: continually setting the bar so high for yourself that you are repeatedly disappointed in yourself. It's the experience of a kid (insert any age here) who, upon getting a 92 or, God forbid, an 84 on an exam views the result as an absolute failure and berates themselves for what they see as their imperfection. There's no room for a story such as "I did pretty well, that was a really hard exam." For Katherine, it didn't matter that she was now performing in a sea of highly talented and superintelligent medical students. She saw her solid class ranking as clear-cut evidence of her own failure—something to be ashamed of and embarrassed by. I've learned from teens that this mindset extends beyond academics to sports and other extracurricular activities. Miss a shot in basketball or commit an error in softball and it feels disastrous. Forget a line in the school play or flub your solo in the a cappella sing-off and the world may as well be ending. Matt, a sophomore cross-country runner, told me that he would beat up on himself for days after posting a poor time in a meet, finding it impossible to escape the recurrent thoughts about his disappointing performance.

Self-oriented maladaptive perfectionism in teens has been a focus of research for at least two decades, and for good reason. It has been found to be associated with depression, anxiety, self-injurious behavior (such as cutting), low self-compassion, and, interestingly and surprisingly to me, bullying. It is also associated with the eating disorder anorexia nervosa and is considered to be one of the psychological forces that is a root cause of this condition. There is clear evidence that rates of self-oriented maladaptive perfectionism in teens and college students have been on the rise in recent decades and that the increase may well be a big part of the reason that rates of depression and anxiety in young people are rising as well.

What Makes Perfectionism Maladaptive

Parents often ask me how to tell if their child has maladaptive perfectionism because, in some ways, it's hard to distinguish from perfectionism—

which is lauded in our society and educational systems. I find that it can be illuminating for parents first to understand how maladaptive perfectionism is measured and then to consider the implications or evidence for their own child—or for themselves.

Self-oriented maladaptive perfectionism can be measured and "diagnosed" with widely used and validated survey instruments. As it isn't an illness, getting a diagnosis isn't possible, which is why I use quotation marks. It's more correct to say that an individual can be classified as having maladaptive perfectionism, but, for me, those words sound a bit cold—dehumanizing even. My favorite tools for measuring the mindset are various forms of the Almost Perfect Scale, first developed in the early 1990s by Robert Slaney,[2] and my preferred choice is the Short Almost Perfect Scale (SAPS).[3] The SAPS consists of two subscales—one for "high standards" and the other for "discrepancy." The high standards subscale, as the name suggests, assesses how high the standards are that people set for themselves, using statements such as "I have high expectations for myself" and "I have a strong need to strive for excellence." The discrepancy subscale assesses the degree to which there is a gap between someone's *desired* performance and their *actual* performance. In other words, it measures their sense of disappointment in themselves when they fall short of their own personal expectations. The discrepancy subscale asks respondents how much they agree with statements like "I am hardly ever satisfied with my performance" and "Doing my best never seems to be enough." If someone scores high on the high standards subscale, they are likely someone who frequently aims for excellence or even perfection. If someone scores high on the discrepancy scale, they experience high levels of disappointment when their performance falls short of their expectations.

In 2020, just before the pandemic, I studied self-oriented maladaptive perfectionism in high schoolers in Ohio and later in college students at SLU.[4] I was interested in seeing how prevalent it was. Using the SAPS high standards subscale, I asked them about their expectations for themselves.

Below is a graph of the scores of the ninth to twelfth graders.

High Standards Subscale

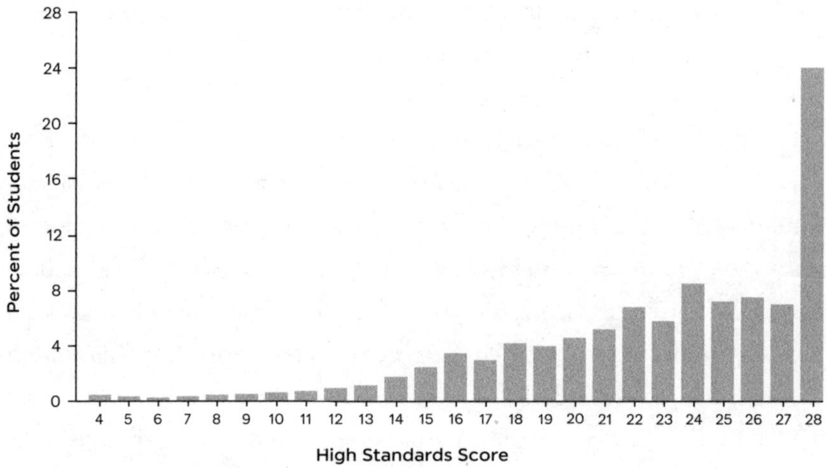

You can see that most students have scores above 23 and almost a quarter have 28, the highest possible score. This means that many of the students set very high standards for themselves—this subscale is related to the character trait "conscientiousness."

This next graph is of SLU college students in an introductory chemistry course.

High Standards Subscale

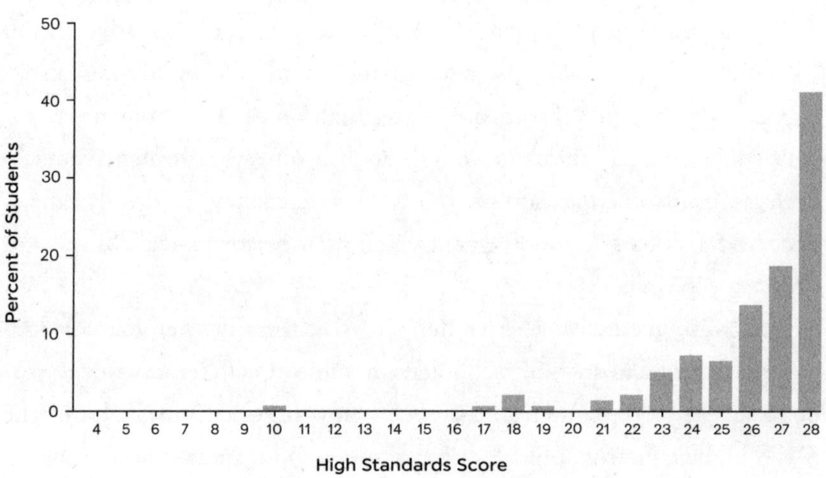

Data adapted from Pfau, Alagic, and Slavin (2024).

Again, we see very high scores on the high standards subscale, higher even than those of the Ohio teenagers, and almost no one scoring low. This means that this group of students set the bar extremely high for themselves.

So, what about the discrepancy subscale? Remember that this one measures someone's sense of disappointment in themselves when their performance falls short of their goals and expectations. A high score on this subscale means high disappointment. Here are the high school students.

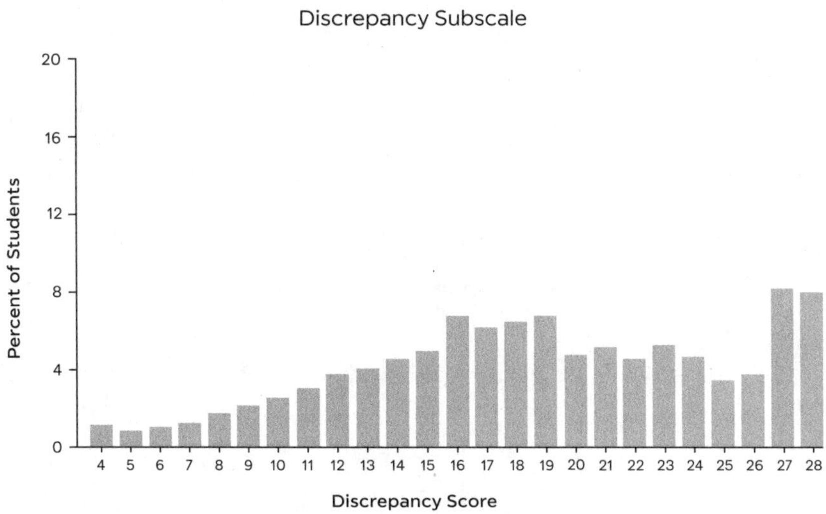

Unlike the cluster of very high scores seen in the high standards subscale, the scores here show a much wider range, though many students still score high. The largest number of students, 8 percent, scored 27 on this scale, meaning that they have a tendency to be very highly disappointed with themselves if they don't achieve their desired goal. On the other hand, a good number of students have scores of ten or lower, meaning that they tend not to get too disappointed with themselves. This might mean that they aim to get an A on a test (high standards) but if they end up with an A minus or a B plus they won't be devastated.

As you can see in the next graph, the college students look similar, although more respondents than the high school students are in the higher ranges, meaning a greater number of them feel disappointed in themselves when they don't reach their goals.

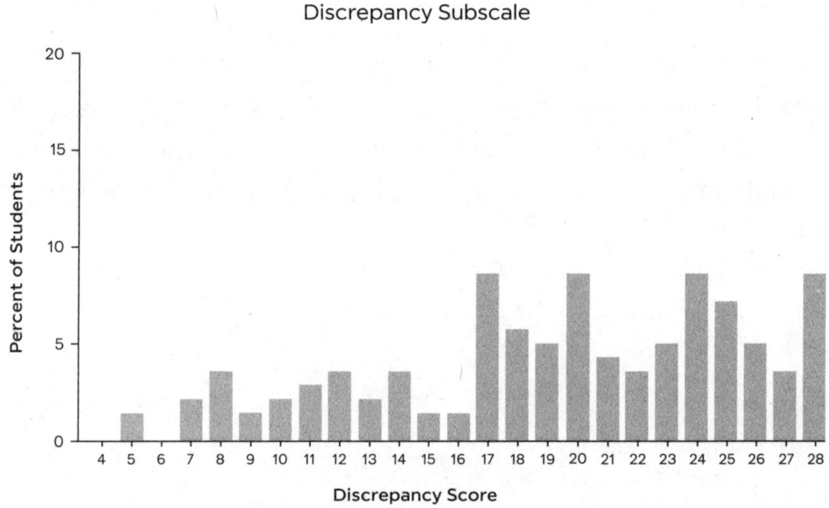

Data adapted from Pfau, Alagic, and Slavin (2024).

So, overall, when we look at these student populations using the data from both the high standards and discrepancy graphs, we see that the great majority are perfectionists, meaning that they have very high standards and set high expectations for themselves. Many of the perfectionists also score high on the discrepancy scale, which means they feel disappointment when they don't meet their own expectations—making them maladaptive perfectionists rather than adaptive perfectionists.

People can show any of four levels, or forms, of self-oriented perfectionism: maladaptive perfectionism, adaptive perfectionism, self-critical nonperfectionism, or satisfied nonperfectionism. Each person can be characterized as one of these types using the scores on the two subscales, as you can see in the following matrix.

	High Standards	Discrepancy
Maladaptive perfectionism	Yes	Yes
Adaptive perfectionism	Yes	No
Self-critical nonperfectionism	No	Yes
Satisfied nonperfectionism	No	No

1. Maladaptive perfectionists (high score on both subscales). This is the child or teen who gets an A minus on an assignment and is devastated. Or the medical student like Katherine who is doing well in school but feels shame because they're not at the top of the class. These kids are often high achievers, but their achievement comes with a price: higher rates of depression and anxiety than any of the other groups. These are the kids who may crack like an egg.

2. Adaptive perfectionists (high score on the high standards subscale, low discrepancy score). These are the kids who strive for high scores or excellence in their extracurricular activities, but they don't beat up on themselves when they fall short. They understand that sometimes you have a bad day, or you studied the wrong section of the material, or maybe you should have gone to bed earlier the night before the test. They accept that perfection isn't possible all the time and are willing to learn from their "imperfection." They tend to have lower rates of depression and anxiety, a higher sense of well-being and life satisfaction, and more positive mood than maladaptive perfectionists. In addition, they usually have

more self-compassion and higher resilience, bouncing back from setbacks more readily than those with maladaptive perfectionism. Interestingly, they are likely to perform better academically too. This lends credence to what we already know but sometimes need to be reminded of: Beating up on yourself does not lead to better performance. These kids are in a sweet spot, managing both to achieve at a high level and to maintain their mental health (as compared to those with maladaptive perfectionism).

3. Self-critical nonperfectionists (low score on the high standards subscale and high discrepancy score). These kids don't shoot for the stars, but they still feel disappointment with themselves when they underdeliver—which can then contribute to poor mental health.

4. Satisfied nonperfectionists (low scores on both subscales). This group includes the kids (most often boys) who don't aim high, are comfortable getting Bs and Cs (or lower) on tests, and prefer to spend their time away from academic endeavors, such as playing videogames. They tend to have better mental health than maladaptive perfectionists, but they may suffer from lower motivation and lower academic achievement.

What Can a Parent Do?

Recognizing Maladaptive Perfectionism in Your Teen

The first important step in addressing maladaptive perfectionism in your child is to be able to recognize it. This may not be as simple as it sounds in a world that values overwork, hyperproductivity, and overachievement, especially if your child is caught up in an educational environment that places excessive demands on students that skew the notion of what is normal.

One way to begin is to ask yourself some questions and see how well they fit your child's behavior. Does your child consistently set very high standards for themselves and have very high personal expectations? Do they often feel disappointed in their own performance even when it seems perfectly fine to you? Are they rarely satisfied with their performance? If your answers to these questions are yes, your child may well suffer from maladaptive perfectionism, and if they are depressed or anxious, this may be contributing to it. Now that you know what maladaptive perfectionism looks like, it can be helpful to observe your child's behavior. Take note of how they behave around studying, homework, and tests in general. Do they seem to put a lot of pressure on themselves to be perfect all the time? What about their extracurriculars? Do they constantly need to win or have the leading role? Keep an eye on their reactions in the wake of a less-than-perfect performance. Do they take in stride a disappointing test score or soccer game, or do they have a full-on meltdown? Or do they perhaps experience something in between, perhaps disappointment and a desire to do better next time, and then move on to the next thing?

You may want to reflect upon your own tendencies toward maladaptive perfectionism and ask yourself if you could be role-modeling self-critical thoughts about yourself or projecting criticism onto your child.

In previous chapters, I introduced you to Emma, a tenth grader with anxiety, and eight-year-old Olivia, who puts herself down if she doesn't get an A. They both suffer from maladaptive perfectionism, which puts enormous pressure on them, leading them to study excessively, get inadequate sleep, experience anxiety before examinations, and, in Emma's case, seek to avoid the stress of school by trying to stay home. For medical student Katherine, this problematic mindset led her to question her own ability, to work even longer hours, and to feel unbearable shame. She was headed in the direction of burnout or breakdown—there's only so long that people can push themselves in the pursuit of impossible goals and bear the brunt of constant feelings of failure.

Sometimes maladaptive perfectionism can show up in other ways:

- Your child shows high levels of anxiety about the possibility of failure.

- They find it hard to take criticism—seeing it as evidence of their "imperfection."
- They redo assignments or constantly start over, convinced their work is not good enough.
- They view mistakes as unacceptable, as signs of weakness.
- They procrastinate, or avoid tasks/schoolwork, to avoid the possibility of failure.
- They are overly critical of themselves and others.
- They don't finish or hand in work because they feel it's not good enough.

Preventing and Managing Maladaptive Perfectionism

It can be hard as a parent to see your child caught in the trap of maladaptive perfectionism. The good news, though, is that it *is not fixed.* It is a learned behavior, one that people can come to recognize and handle. Importantly, as a parent, you can take concrete steps to prevent it from developing and to manage it if your child is already caught in its snare.

Keep the pressure off. A primary goal as a parent is to not engage in other-oriented perfectionism, such as insisting that your child bring home perfect grades, always ace the test, or be on the winning team. Your child already feels the weight of stress and pressure so prevalent outside the home—and there is no need for you to add to it. Pressure in school starts much earlier than high school, often beginning in elementary school. When you chat with your child after school, ask how their day went or about friends and activities, rather than homing in on test results.

Notice the effort they put in. Praise effort before the big game or test, but not too effusively. "I noticed how hard you've been working on your test prep." If your child does get stellar grades, you can say you are proud of them, with the emphasis on the effort expended and what they learned from the experience. Make sure it is clear to them that your love is not contingent upon their performance.

Consider your own perfectionist tendencies. Listen to what you say about your own performance, your own successes and failures. How do you process those in front of your kids? Try to embrace mistakes and failure and help your child see the value in learning from what didn't go as planned. When your kid falls short of their own expectations, you can point to your own failures and say that you're doing just fine despite these trip-ups. Also, if you have a spouse or partner, how do you react when they make a mistake, when they are late, when they forget to run an errand? Aim to show patience and compassion in those situations rather than frustration, disappointment, and recrimination. Your child is watching and listening.

Managing a maladaptive perfectionism meltdown: If your child is breaking down because of some disappointing performance, whether on an exam or in an extracurricular activity like a sport, you can use the basic steps that I introduced in chapter 3:

1. **Validate their thoughts.** "I know how hard you worked for this exam, and I can understand that you are disappointed."
2. **Empathize with their feelings.** "Given the pressure in school to do well, I can understand why this would feel so distressing."
3. **Probe for understanding.** "Is there something deeper that you're worried about other than just the score?" Their response to this will guide your answer and may involve challenging their negative self-talk using cognitive restructuring. This technique can help them recognize the distorted mindsets and thoughts they are experiencing and construct a different, more accurate and self-compassionate narrative. I will describe this approach in the next chapter.

As you're already probably aware, kids can often discount or outright reject the wisdom a parent offers, but don't give up in the face of this resistance! Keep saying things like "No one is perfect," "We all make mistakes," or "I care more about your effort and what you are learning than what your score is." Over time, they will come to know your values and begin to incorporate them gradually into their own thoughts.

Impostor Phenomenon

The next problematic mindset that we are going to examine is impostor phenomenon. It is just what it sounds like: feeling like an impostor, or a fraud, believing that any success you've had is due to sheer luck, and believing that you're not as smart and capable as people think you are. You've been fooling others all along, and it's only a matter of time before they figure this out and see the true you. This self-doubt can lead to harsh self-criticism. Some use the term *impostor syndrome,* but to me that sounds like a disease that may be difficult to cure. I prefer *phenomenon,* which sounds more ephemeral, more easily changed—which it is—and more like something that can happen *to* you rather than something that *is* you.

Impostor phenomenon is often experienced by high-achieving, objectively successful people, including teens and young adults who seem to be doing very well in school. It has been found to be associated with depression, anxiety, low self-esteem, maladaptive perfectionism, overwork, and burnout, and at times it can contribute to lower academic performance.[5] In some cases, it leads teens to overexert themselves, throwing themselves into endless hours of studying in an effort to prove themselves worthy of success, though often it can lead to paralysis or underperformance as teens start to view their efforts as futile.

Impostor phenomenon is not consistently present. It can simmer along and lessen as you become more confident in an academic or work situation, but it can also flare, often during periods of transition, particularly in academic environments—from elementary to middle school, middle school to high school, high school to college, and college to graduate school—

and can contribute to significant distress. Surges in expectations and demands that often accompany these transitions fuel the reappearance of impostor phenomenon. Perhaps the most difficult transition can occur between high school and college, particularly for students who are admitted to highly selective colleges and suddenly find themselves surrounded by students who are just as smart if not smarter.

Our medical student Katherine struggled with impostor phenomenon along with maladaptive perfectionism in her first year of medical school, her solid but average performance leading her to doubt her own academic ability and to live in fear of being exposed for the fraud she thought she was. Over time, she learned how to manage these problematic mindsets, but she experienced a severe flare in the first months of residency training after medical school. She described to me her feelings of "terror" whenever she clicked on the button to enter medical orders for patients, convinced that she was incompetent and could cause people harm. Katherine recovered from that bout of impostorism, ultimately thriving in residency, and she is now a faculty member in ophthalmology. Her journey is a good reminder that impostor phenomenon is not fixed, that it can ease as you become more comfortable in a role, and that there are effective tools for its management.

The Effect of Environment on Impostor Phenomenon

It's important to note that impostor phenomenon is not only an internal construct. The environment can contribute significantly to feelings of impostorism, something I acutely realized a number of years ago. A SLU medical graduate, a truly extraordinary young Black woman, had gone off to an internship in general surgery in a program on the East Coast. I had served as an informal mentor to her during medical school, and she was among my favorite students. She reached out to me a few months into her intern year to say she would be visiting St. Louis soon, and could we meet for coffee? I enthusiastically agreed. When we met, I of course wanted to know how her residency was going, as surgery is notoriously rigorous and demanding. She said that she was doing well. I went on to ask her if she had experienced impostor feelings, and she answered immediately, "Every day." I was floored. I had never before heard this answer.

"What do you mean, every day?"

"Every day I'm *made* to feel like I'm an impostor, that as a young Black woman, I'm not supposed to be a surgeon. It's patients, nurses, faculty, residents, everyone."

As a white man, across my forty-plus years in academic medicine, I had *never once* been made to feel like I didn't belong. So, as we consider these mindsets, we need to remember that the environment we exist in, the systems and power structures, can make you feel that you are an impostor and punish or discount you for perceived deficits. These experiences can be shaped, influenced, and amplified by a whole host of factors, such as race, ethnicity, gender, sexual orientation, and disability. For example, a girl in a math class may feel like she is not supposed to do well, conditioned in part by internalizing math-gender stereotypes, and when she does do well she may feel like it was just luck. Black students in a gifted program may feel like they don't belong there if every time they raise their hand in class, teachers call on white students instead.

What Can a Parent Do?

Recognizing Impostor Phenomenon in Your Child

The term *impostor phenomenon* was originally coined by two psychologists, Drs. Pauline Clance and Suzanne Imes, in 1978 in their landmark study of high-achieving women.[6] Importantly, they developed a survey instrument, the Clance Impostor Phenomenon Scale (CIPS),[7] which measures impostor phenomenon and continues to garner widespread use. A number of other instruments exist, including the Leary Impostorism Scale (LIS), which I have used in my research.[8] As with maladaptive perfectionism, the first step in helping your child with impostor phenomenon is to be able to recognize it. Using concepts underlying the various impostorism scales can be helpful in that process. Think about your child and their behavior. Are they frequently afraid that they will fail in a new assignment or an upcoming exam even if they generally perform well? Do they feel like their success is primarily due to luck? Are they afraid that others' high opinions of them are unfounded and that their true self will be discovered at some point; are they afraid that they have only been fooling people?

Notice the number of times the word *afraid* comes up. Impostor phenomenon is, in many ways, rooted in fear: fear of failure that can lead to overpreparation or, alternatively, procrastination; fear of being "found out" that can contribute to self-doubt and anxiety; and, particularly in first-generation students and racial and ethnic minority groups in elite high schools and colleges, fear that can be associated with feelings of being undeserving.

Parents can also look out for the following signs:

- Persistent self-doubt despite success
- Intense fear of failure
- Overwork
- Procrastination or avoidance
- Downplaying successes or achievements
- Avoidance of new activities
- A dislike or dismissal of compliments

Preventing and Managing Impostor Phenomenon

If your child makes statements or voices feelings consistent with impostor phenomenon, again use the steps of validating their concerns, empathizing with their feelings, and probing for understanding. These additional steps can also be helpful:

Don't overpraise or praise as a matter of course. Many adults with impostor phenomenon were praised for every little thing when they were children and were made to feel as if they were extraordinary in everything they did. Once they were out in the world, they found that this just wasn't accurate, and they began to question all the compliments they had received as a child. Was any of it true, and, if not, were they good at anything at all?

Praise effort, not outcome. When you praise the effort that your child puts into a project, whether schoolwork or their hobbies, you help them see that there is a process at play that is important, one that takes time and involves their own hard work and commitment. Over time they connect the dots between their effort and the outcome, and they can see evidence of their own role in the work, helping to counter feelings of being a fraud.

Be realistic and honest. Help your kids get a picture of their strengths and weaknesses, rather than leading them to believe that they are excellent across the board. It can be helpful for them to see where they can improve, what is difficult for them, and what comes naturally.

Keep a success log. Kids with impostor phenomenon often only remember their failures and then use them as evidence that they are a fraud. If you encourage them to compile evidence of things they've done well, it will be hard to dispute. Remember to define success as more than an outcome. Their log might include helping to housetrain the family puppy, supporting a classmate who was in distress, or finishing their science project even though they found it difficult.

It's also important to say that impostor phenomenon isn't a binary, something that you have or you don't. Like the other mindsets, it exists on a continuum. Dr. Eric Nadel, a physician at Massachusetts General Hospital, once shared an insight that I carry with me today. He said, "The opposite of impostor is not no impostor, it's arrogance." And the corollary to that is that having a bit of impostor is probably good; it involves some humility and some self-questioning, will lead to fewer rash decisions or mistakes born of overconfidence, and will likely make you a more pleasant person to be around.

In the next chapter, I'll help you with responses to try to counter the messages your child is telling themselves, to change their maladaptive mindset and help them see the world and themselves through a different lens.

Performance as Identity

This mindset is one that I first became aware of in conversations with my daughters and with medical students at SLU. It is characterized, for example, by thoughts after receiving a disappointing score on an exam such as "I *am* that score" rather than "I *got* that score": In other words, the score is a measure of your worth and value as a human being rather than an assessment of that particular performance. This was a trap that our sophomore student Emma fell into, intersecting with her maladaptive perfectionism to compound the pain. She wasn't just disappointed in her performance when she got less than a perfect score; she was disappointed with *herself*, a much more distressing experience. Performance as identity is part of a larger construct—contingent self-worth—a critically important developmental feature of adolescence in which one's self-worth is tied to positive external feedback (such as grades, wins, and compliments) in areas such as academics, sports, one's social world, one's appearance. In a society that prioritizes achievement, it isn't surprising that countless numbers of young people tie their self-worth to how well they perform in any or all of these arenas.

In my research in high schools and with medical students, I didn't use formal scales to assess performance as identity; instead I asked a single telling question: *To what degree is your self-worth tied to your own self-imposed standards of academic performance?* Students could choose from five responses: not at all, slightly, moderately, very much, a great deal.

In the schools I studied, approximately 75 percent of students answered moderately or higher. This mindset is widespread and only increasing as societal, parental, and kids' own expectations rise. In my surveys, I found that overall, the higher teens scored on this question, the higher their depression and anxiety scores. It's possible that performance as identity feels good when you're on top of the heap, but when your performance is less than what you wish it to be (which can be much of the time if you're striving for perfection), the negative impact on your mental health and well-being can be substantial. One research study looking at performance-based self-esteem in medical students linked it to burnout.[9]

Performance as identity can also lead to a fear of failure, excessive distress in the face of setbacks, and a narrowing of interests and activities as more and more energy is channeled into keeping up performance in specific categories such as academics, sports, or one's standing on social media.

What Can a Parent Do?

Recognizing Performance as Identity in Your Child

This mindset is fairly easy to spot as kids tend to use "I am . . ." statements rather than "I did" or "I got." Typical performance-as-identity statements include "I'm so stupid," "I'm such an idiot," or "I'm a loser," instead of "I did badly on the test" or "I messed up during practice."

Other signs include:

- Over-reliance on external validation, whether from people or from social media "likes"
- Self-esteem tied up in outcomes, so that one's mood rises and falls based on performance
- Difficulty in bouncing back after less-than-perfect performances
- Fear of failure, which can lead to procrastination or paralysis
- Hyperfocus on academics (or sports/social/appearance) to the detriment of other aspects of life

Preventing and Managing Performance as Identity

Don't overemphasize the importance of performance. One of the most influential things that you can do as a parent is to pull back from focusing on scores and achievement, and especially don't make your child feel like your love and approval is contingent on high scores or successful performances. It can be hard not to do so as we've all been instilled with the idea of success as winning or being at the top. But when we focus primarily on how our child did—rather than who they are—we can contribute to and reinforce thoughts of performance as identity, touching off a toxic cycle of increased performance pressure, fear of failure, and lowered self-esteem when performance doesn't meet expectations.

Develop an interest in broader aspects of your child's life. Many of us have the tendency to ask how the exam went as soon as our child walks through the door. If you catch yourself doing that, try to curb the habit. You can ask later or, better yet, wait until your child brings it up, if they do. If your child shares with you that they got an excellent result on their history test or scored the winning point in their volleyball game, you can certainly praise them, but add that you've been impressed by their hard work throughout the semester and that they seemed to have learned a lot or made good progress. This could be followed by a question about what they found most interesting in their study or on which of their teammates were playing that day, turning the focus to what they learned or the collective team effort rather than their score.

Make your home a nonjudgment zone. Send the message that performances are not always stellar (they cannot be) but that your child is always loved. If your child brings home a disappointing grade on an English paper or tells you they made an error in their baseball game, don't add to the judgment they are feeling themselves. Move to a place of compassion instead.

Stay away from the school electronic dashboard. Many schools now have an electronic dashboard or digital portal through which parents have constant and often real-time access to their child's academic performance (including quiz, test, and exam scores as well as a running GPA). It is easy to fall into the trap of repeatedly checking for scores—and then commenting on them to your child, heightening their awareness that this is an important focus for you. If you find this is something that you do, try to limit checking scores to once a week or less, and to hold back on conversations with your teen about what you have seen there. Eli, a teen in a school near Portland, Maine, told me how much pressure it added, knowing that his parents were constantly checking his grades. He felt like he was wearing a sign around his neck with his current GPA. Often he avoided conversations with his parents as he knew they would bring up his latest test results.

Take steps to help your child develop multiple identities. Rather than your child having a singular identity tied to their performance in academics, sports, or other activities, help them cultivate richer identities that can include artistic ability, creative thinking, compassion for others, kindness, and trustworthiness, to name a few examples. Look for opportunities to praise these attributes so that praise about successful performances isn't the only kind that they hear. In chapter 7, we'll further explore this approach of broadening your child's interests and goals as part of a discussion of goal disruption theory.

Not everything is a performance. Help your child understand that not everything we do needs to be a performance of some kind, or tied to success or failure. For example, being a grandchild and visiting their grandparents for dinner brings joy and connection; finding a new series of books that they love might develop their identity as a curious book lover.

Consider what you're modeling. Is your sense of self-worth caught up in your work? Do you tend to think of your success in life as related to your career? Try to emphasize other areas of your identity to your kids—maybe you love to listen to jazz or build model airplanes or you're a member of the local school board. Let them know how much these other aspects of your identity mean to you. Think about how you describe other people to your kids—do you say, "She's the top neurosurgeon in New York" or "He went to Harvard," or do you lead with "You'll really like her. She loves the ocean too," or "Ask him about the time he saw a rattlesnake." These are subtle ways you can change how your kids see the world—and themselves.

In the next chapter, we'll look at specific approaches that your child can use when performance as identity arises in their everyday life and they hear the self-critical voice that tells them they're stupid or a loser.

Toxic Comparison

Toxic comparison is another common mindset, especially prevalent among teens and college students, and developing in younger kids too. It can manifest in a couple of ways: feeling good about yourself only when you are outcompeting others; and, inversely, feeling bad about yourself when you constantly compare yourself to others and find yourself lacking, whether in school performance, social status, or appearance. For some kids, being above average in school is good enough, but others may feel content only if they are in the top 5 or 10 percent, and some are satisfied only if they are the valedictorian of their class. Medical student Katherine was suffering from toxic comparison when she came to meet with me, but you don't have to be a stressed-out medical student to fall into this harmful mindset. A mom shared the story of her fifteen-year-old daughter, Maddie, who was in a high-achieving high school in Chicago. No matter how well Maddie did in her schoolwork, she was always miserable because she continually assessed her performance in relation to that of the other kids in her class. If Maddie got a 94 on a test, there was always someone who had achieved a 95. And it didn't stop with academics. It rippled outward to her clothing, her appearance, her friendships, until she was dissatisfied with every aspect of her life. Her self-esteem plummeted. Toxic comparison can be magnified and compounded by social media, where we are constantly comparing ourselves to other people and falling far short—usually forgetting that we are only seeing the curated and filtered highlights of their lives while we are living in the ongoing chaos of our own.

What Can a Parent Do?

Recognizing Toxic Comparison in Your Child

Toxic comparison may start in childhood—no surprise, given the continual testing that begins so early in schooling. Kids know from elementary school that they are being measured, sorted, and ranked, and that those rankings matter. As a consequence, they may start to feel good about themselves only if they are performing better than their classmates and, inversely, may struggle when they perceive themselves as inadequate. This early social conditioning paves the way for a lifetime of evaluating themselves in relation to others, which affects how they view their self-worth.

Toxic comparison can be spotted fairly easily. Statements tend to fall into a couple of categories. First are those in which children specifically compare themselves to others. "Justin is so much smarter than me!" "Stella is so much more popular than I am." They can also manifest in goal setting that is based on outperforming others rather than personal achievements. "I'm gonna crush Mack in tennis today!" "I'll show Janie! She's not going to get gold today."

Other signs include:

- Low self-esteem, which may lead to social withdrawal
- Frequent self-criticism and putting oneself down
- Focus on failures and shortcomings rather than seeing the full complement of one's attributes and achievements
- Anxiety and worry about performance
- Being overly competitive with peers and needing to constantly "win"

It can be heartbreaking to see your child caught in the trap of toxic comparison, especially as you can see how special they are and how many strengths they have. When Maddie's mom told a friend that her daughter pretty much hated every aspect of herself and thought that everyone else was better than her, her friend was astonished. "Maddie!?" she said. "But she's amazing! I love being around her—she's funny and smart and kind. I can hardly believe that!"

Show unconditional love. Your child needs your support. Now is not the time for criticism or judgment. Instead of saying, "How can you think that about yourself?" keep going with a constant refrain of caring statements. "Thanks for making me laugh—I was feeling down and you know how to cheer me up." "What a great idea for your science project. I can't wait to see what you do with it."

Your child is unique. Remind your child that they have many strengths and skills, that they are a unique person. You'll learn in chapter 7 how to encourage your child to develop multiple identities, and this is a circumstance where you can reinforce that. You can use statements that highlight their different dimensions: "We can't always outdo everyone in everything we do, but I love all of the qualities and skills that you have—your kindness, your creativity, your compassion."

They can't always be the best. Let them know that there is more to life than being the winner, the leader, or the best at everything, and emphasize your appreciation of effort and your pride in many aspects of their lives.

Share stories from your own life. It can help to say how you have felt inadequate sometimes but learned and thrived even though you weren't number one. A friend of mine told his son that two of his colleagues had gotten awards at work and that he was initially disappointed. After thinking about it, he decided it was better to be happy for his colleagues and celebrate their success, and continue to work hard and try to improve.

The Relationship of Feelings and Emotions to Maladaptive Mindsets

Maybe you have recognized some or all of these mindsets in your child and can begin to see how these cognitive processes profoundly influence the narratives that many kids construct about themselves. It's also important to note that these mindsets can bring forth certain emotions, such as feelings of inadequacy, embarrassment, and shame, which can exacerbate distress and are strongly correlated with depression and anxiety. My initial conversation with medical student Katherine sparked my interest in studying maladaptive mindsets as well as the feelings that seemed to spring from them, specifically the shame that she experienced. To explore this phenomenon further, Katherine and I decided to conduct a study (for which she was ultimately lead author) of medical students at SLU examining the relationship of maladaptive perfectionism and impostor phenomenon to feelings of inadequacy, embarrassment, and shame, and also to depression and anxiety.[10] The findings were clear and striking. Students (like Katherine) who screened positive for maladaptive perfectionism or impostor phenomenon were much more likely to harbor feelings of inadequacy, embarrassment, and/or shame. And those who felt inadequacy, embarrassment, and/or shame were much more likely to screen positive for depression and anxiety.

The study did not prove that maladaptive perfectionism and impostor phenomenon cause depression and anxiety; it could only show that there is an association between maladaptive perfectionism and impostor phenomenon and these mental health outcomes. However, for decades cognitive psychologists have believed, supported by numerous research studies, that negative thoughts can contribute to negative feelings and that those negative feelings can contribute to adverse mental health outcomes. Our study was consistent with a large body of previous research. Since that study of medical students, I have continued to explore these negative emotions in high school and college populations and have found strong correlations of feelings of inadequacy, embarrassment, and shame with depression and anxiety.

This chapter may have been eye-opening for many of you, as these problematic mindsets are widespread and insidious in the damage that they can cause, yet are often overlooked. In many instances, particularly in our success-based society, we accept them as normal. If this chapter hit close to home for your child (or for you), there is hope. The techniques that I have shared throughout this chapter will alleviate your child's distress in many ways, but in the next chapter I'll go one step further. The problematic mindsets can be changed, and I'll provide you with specific techniques to empower your child to challenge and overcome the distorted worldview that the mindsets help shape.

Chapter 6

Cognitive Distortions: How Unhelpful Thoughts Can Amplify Distress

It's 10:00 p.m. and Alex, a sixteen-year-old high school sophomore, is crying as he sits at the kitchen table doing homework. His mother walks in, her brow furrowed in concern, and asks, "What's wrong?" Between sobs, Alex says, "I looked at the dashboard and I got an 87 on my math quiz!" "Oh, honey," says his mom, putting her hand on his shoulder, "I'm sure you'll do better next time." "But you don't understand! This means I won't get an A in this course and my GPA is going to drop. And now I'll never get into Carnegie Mellon! Or work for Google!" The mother looks at her distraught son, worried and surprised by his reaction. "You don't know that for sure," she offers. "But it's true," says Alex. "Everybody says so!" And he storms off to his bedroom, slamming the door.

You may have seen this scenario, or some version of it, play out with your own kids, and while it may seem overdramatic or even absurd at times, it's important to pay attention to the behavior as it can be a sign of significant distress in your child. Alex was experiencing a common cognitive distortion called catastrophizing—predicting a disastrous future outcome that will inevitably occur because of a single, often relatively small event. In his case, that one disappointing math test result would usher in a series of terrible future outcomes for him. Cognitive distortions can be thought of as a collection of microreactions—automatic, often unhelpful, thoughts triggered by unexpected events or situations, frequently leading to inaccurate interpretations of reality and reinforcing negative thinking. Ultimately, they tend to make us feel bad about ourselves. They are incredibly common and can intersect with the demands and pressures of achievement culture to produce severe upset and dysfunction for kids and parents alike.

I'll begin this chapter by introducing these cognitive traps and describe how they can negatively affect kids, especially teens, their disruptive effects rippling out in their (and our) lives. I'll provide definitions, descriptions, and examples of each of the most common distortions that I've observed as a clinician, educator, and researcher to help you identify them:

- Magnification
- All-or-nothing thinking
- Personalization and self-blame
- Overgeneralization
- Tunnel vision
- Fortune-telling
- Catastrophizing
- Mind reading
- Disbelief

It's important to note that cognitive distortions frequently appear together and often go hand in hand with problematic mindsets, feeding and reinforcing one another. The good news is that an effective solution exists that works for both: cognitive restructuring. I'll describe this empowering technique to help you and your child recognize when they are using these unhelpful mindsets or distortions and to learn how to manage them—and even to stop them in their tracks.

Understanding Cognitive Distortions

Cognitive distortions were first described by Aaron Beck, the psychiatrist who developed cognitive behavioral therapy, whom I introduced in chapter 3.[1] In his research, Beck noticed that many of his depressed patients had distorted thinking patterns that, he believed, contributed to their mental illness. He wrote, "He [the depressed patient] tends to perceive his present, future, and the outside world (the cognitive triad) in a negative way and consequently shows a biased interpretation of his experiences, negative expectancies as to the probable success of anything he undertakes, and a massive amount of self-criticism."[2]

This idea of distorted thought patterns and their connection to distress has long roots. In the Western world, it can be traced to Stoicism, an early Greek school of thought founded in the third century BCE, and in Eastern thought, to Buddhism, which dates to the sixth century BCE in India. Stoic philosopher Epictetus (ca. 50–135 CE) wrote, "Men are disturbed not by things, but by the views which they take of things,"[3] while Roman emperor Marcus Aurelius, in his magnum opus, *Meditations* (ca. 170–180 CE), stated, "If you are distressed by anything external, the pain is not due to the thing itself but to your estimate of it; and this you have the power to revoke at any moment."[4]

Similarly, a well-known Buddhist teaching holds that when something bad happens, two arrows fly at us. The first arrow is the incident itself, and the trajectory and impact of that arrow cannot be changed; it will hit and lead to pain. However, the second arrow represents the *meaning* that we attach to the event, the thoughts and beliefs that rise up after the first arrow strikes. Buddhist monk and peace activist Thich Nhat Hanh taught that this second arrow not only may add to the pain caused by the first arrow but can multiply it. He advised not to exaggerate its importance, stating, "If you stop to worry, to be fearful, to protest, to be angry about the pain, then you magnify the pain ten times or more. Your worry is the second arrow. You should protect yourself and not allow the second arrow to come, because the second arrow comes from you."[5]

In the 1960s, Beck categorized five primary distortions that he had noticed, also referring to them as "automatic thoughts," and he added two more to his list in 1979. His initial names for the various distortions reflected his academic roots and included less-than-catchy terms such as *arbitrary inference* and *selective abstraction,* which were hard for the layperson to understand. However, David D. Burns, a psychiatrist and student of Beck, popularized more familiar names for each of the cognitive distortions in his bestselling book *Feeling Good: The New Mood Therapy,* published in 1980, and brought them into more general awareness. Those are the terms that I'll use in this chapter and throughout the book.

The Impact on Daily Life

Cognitive distortions can be experienced by all of us. As I introduce them, many will likely seem familiar and you'll remember incidents and situations where you have used them. However, they are strongly associated with depression and anxiety, as well as other mental health illnesses, including anorexia nervosa, panic disorder, and borderline personality disorder, meaning that people with these conditions are more prone to cognitive distortions. One recent study in which people self-reported a diagnosis of depression found that their language on social media was characterized by higher levels of distorted thinking compared to a random sample.[6] Interestingly, much of the evidence to support the importance of cognitive distortions in depression and anxiety is indirect, seen through the improvement of symptoms when people are able to employ tools acquired in cognitive behavioral therapy to recognize and manage their problematic mindsets and distortions.

Even when a mental health condition is not present, cognitive distortions can contribute to deep emotional distress that can disrupt young people's lives, leading to strained friendships, difficult family relationships, avoidance and withdrawal, reduced motivation, low self-esteem, physical health issues, and the development of the anxiety dependence trap.

The Distortions

Depending on where you look or whom you talk to, you'll find different lists of diverse cognitive distortions with varying names. Over the years, as I've worked with teens, young adults, medical students, parents, and colleagues, I've compiled my own list of the ones that feel most salient to me.

Magnification: Taking a relatively small event and blowing it up into something huge. It's the experience of getting a disappointing score on a quiz that represents only 5 percent of the final grade for a course and feeling like it's a complete disaster. Magnification is not limited to academic performance but can rear its head in all aspects of life. Julia, a junior in high school, has a number of close friends, but a somewhat difficult conversation with one of them makes her feel criticized and she comes home in a flood of tears. In football, Chris feels like he didn't perform well during practice and is furious with himself, letting his dark mood dominate the rest of his day, even though this is just one of fifty practices the team has during the season.

All-or-Nothing Thinking: This distortion, also known as black-and-white thinking, is strongly connected to maladaptive perfectionism and often acts in concert with magnification. While magnification has to do with the importance or size of the event that caused the distress, all-or-nothing thinking is related to the nature of the outcome. If something isn't completely successful—a test result, a presentation, an interview—then it's an absolute failure. For a high school baseball player, all-or-nothing thinking can lead to profound distress when they make an error in a game; for a dancer, one misstep during a recital becomes a catastrophic event. Kids who struggle with this distortion view outcomes as black and white; there are no grays. There is no room for a thought like "I did pretty well" or the idea that everyone makes mistakes at times. This rigid, inflexible thinking often leads to harsh self-judgment and self-criticism.

Personalization and Self-Blame: When things don't go well, there can be a tendency to assign blame to something or someone. With this cognitive distortion, someone places all the blame on themselves, even when there is no reason to do so. After receiving a disappointing score on a test, the person thinks, "How could I be so stupid? I should have studied more!" rather than "That was a difficult test. It included material we hadn't been taught!" When Michelle's soccer team loses a close game, she sees herself as the person responsible for the outcome rather than acknowledging it as a collective failure. Even when her teammates tell her it's not the case, she insists that's she's the weak link, the reason for the loss, and that they'd be better off without her. Personalization and self-blame don't take into account external factors or events beyond one's control. A teen might blame themselves for their parents' divorce or for a friend getting bullied even though they're likely not responsible for either outcome. That said, willingness to take on a little self-blame is healthy, especially for those who tend to deflect blame from themselves and place it on others. Balance is the key here: taking accountability for your actions, without being excessively and unnecessarily self-critical.

Overgeneralization: This distortion involves taking a single negative event and viewing it as part of an inevitable set pattern of negative things you *always* do or that *always* happen to you. Falling out with a friend can lead to thoughts or beliefs such as "No one likes me! I don't know why I bother trying to make friends!" Or doing poorly on a history test can be followed by statements like "I never do well on these tests," even when you've performed well previously. When Savannah didn't get an interview after applying for a summer internship at a local museum, she was convinced that no one would *ever* hire her. Overgeneralization can lead to negative self-talk and low self-esteem. Ultimately, it can cause someone to always assume the worst, to predict future negative outcomes and give up before they've even tried. "I *always* miss penalty kicks, so I just won't take any."

Tunnel Vision: Focusing on a single negative event—or only the negative aspects of an event—and discounting anything positive in the event or in your life. With this distortion, it's as if nothing can enter your field of perception except this one bad thing, causing you to ignore the good. If you play a less-than-stellar tennis match, all you can see is that single disappointing match, not all the times that you have performed well. You also miss the couple of aces you served in one of the games or the way you kept striving in the face of defeat. When a high school student with tunnel vision performs at less than their usual level in a science course, they lose sight of all the times they've performed at a high level on quizzes and exams. Teens often find themselves homing in on their teacher's one critical piece of feedback, forgetting or ignoring the multiple positive comments, or remembering their friend's insensitive text instead of their dozens of supportive and caring ones. Seeing the world through the distortion of tunnel vision can reinforce negative beliefs and lead to self-doubt and low self-esteem.

Fortune-Telling: Those who experience this cognitive distortion predict a negative future outcome with certainty. It's not simply worrying about a possible bad outcome but rather being sure that one will occur. It was not unusual for my older daughter to tell me that she was going to fail an exam in high school. When I would invariably point out to her that she had never failed one before, she insisted, "This one's different!" Like the other distortions, fortune-telling is not just seen with schoolwork but can appear in essentially any setting. For teens it can often involve their performance, whether on the debate team, in a field hockey game, or in the marching band. It can also be seen with social situations. Beliefs or statements such as "No one is going to talk to me at this party," "I'm never going to have a girlfriend," or "I'm going to have a terrible time in camp this summer" are driven by fortune-telling. When the outcome is already known, there is little room for thinking of strategies or approaches to improve a situation. This can sometimes lead to fortune-telling statements coming true—the self-fulfilling prophecy—thereby reinforcing the cycle.

Catastrophizing: Taking an event or situation (sometimes minor) and believing that it (or a series of ensuing consequences) will end with a future catastrophic outcome. Worry can spin out of control and become disproportionate to the event in question. Alex, our teen with a disappointing score on his math quiz, was experiencing this distortion. Instead of only worrying about how his score would affect his near future (i.e., his grade in the class), he was catastrophizing, believing that it would cause a cascade of circumstances and lead to the worst-possible outcomes—keeping him from being accepted to his dream college and getting his ideal job. A premedical student in an introductory chemistry course stuck firmly to her belief that one quiz score would result in her never getting into medical school or having a fulfilling career. A high school senior, when asked what her top choice for college was, answered Stanford. When asked what she'd do if she didn't get in, she said, "I'll never be happy." It's easy to see how this tendency to always jump to the most extreme, negative outcome can cause unnecessary worry, which can lead to heightened anxiety.

Mind Reading: Believing, with certainty, that you know what someone is thinking, or why they are behaving in a particular way, without having any real evidence. It's the experience of a tenth grader encountering a friend walking toward them at school; the friend looks up briefly, frowns, then looks back down without saying hello. And what does the student believe? *I must have done something to offend them and they're mad at me.* We all experience this cognitive distortion to some extent. When there's a delay in answers to emails or texts, we believe that someone is angry with us (or is feeling one of many negative emotions toward us). Maybe they are, but do we stop to examine the evidence? Or to consider alternatives—that their parent or beloved pet might be sick, or they just had an argument with a friend, or they have a migraine headache, or any number of potential reasons that could account for their behavior? Why are we so sure that we know what they are thinking? In other common situations, teens may believe that everyone thinks they're boring or a loser, so they'll sit alone at lunch; or they may believe that their teacher thinks they're stupid, so they'll stop raising their hand to answer questions in class.

Disbelief: When someone tries to talk you out of irrational or unhelpful thoughts, you simply discount their reasoning as false. Parents know this one well. It's an unwillingness to listen when someone points out the flaws in your thinking. Instead, you dismiss the witness as untrustworthy.

When Alex's mom gently suggested to him the next day that his math score likely wouldn't affect his admission to Carnegie Mellon—and that there were other schools that he would enjoy—he rejected her words. "You're just saying this because you love me and don't want me to be sad!" Disbelief doesn't only occur with external voices; it can exist within your own thoughts too. It can lead to the rejection of evidence that your thought process is incorrect. For example, you might believe that you're bad at physics, and when you get a strong score on a physics exam, you might discount your success by thinking you just got lucky.

Many of us experience problematic mindsets and cognitive distortions on occasion, but when they are pervasive and frequent they can severely affect someone's life and make it hard for them to function. If we return to Emma's story, which I first introduced in chapter 3, we can see how they contributed to her breakdown during her sophomore year. Her anxiety was rooted in the *intersection* of her mindsets and distortions with academic and extracurricular demands and pressure, each exacerbating the other, leading to a cycle of extreme distress. The primary mindset that Emma experienced was maladaptive perfectionism. It contributed to her anxiety and attempted school avoidance by causing her to pursue perfect grades while increasing her worry about not achieving them. This, in turn, prompted a desire to avoid school, the source of her distress. It had other impacts as well. It led her to overstudy, keeping her up late at night and producing chronic sleep deficits that impaired her cognitive and emotional functioning.

Whenever Emma received less-than-perfect scores on quizzes or exams, she experienced multiple cognitive distortions: She magnified and engaged in all-or-nothing thinking, fortune-telling, and catastrophizing, believing that her college hopes were dashed and her future was bleak. Any mistakes that she made during volleyball were met with similar distortions, and when her team lost she blamed herself. Her meltdowns in response to perceived academic and sporting failures repeatedly activated her fight-or-flight mechanism and bathed her system in cortisol and all its negative short- and long-term consequences. She was frequently irritable with her parents, who, acting as mental health first responders, were stressed and exhausted, feeling incapable of adequately supporting Emma. Their repeated rescues pushed them further into the anxiety-dependence trap. Emma's resilience, rather than growing with experiences of adversity, was waning. Her parents were doing their best to support her, but it wasn't enough.

Fortunately, as she made her way through her sophomore year, Emma began to work with a therapist using cognitive behavioral therapy, and hopefully it will help turn the tide for her. She learned the same strategies and approaches to address her mindsets and distortions that we will go through next—and that you can use as you engage with your child and try to best support them by ultimately empowering them to help themselves. Let me reiterate at the outset, however, that if your child has significant symptoms of depression or anxiety, this kind of support is not a substitute for mental health care by a professional. For advice on finding a therapist, see page 64.

What Can a Parent Do?

Parents can take an active role in helping their child recognize and then manage their problematic mindsets and distortions using the tool of cognitive restructuring. In the pages that follow, I'll walk you through the basics of this effective method so that you and your child can turn to it when necessary.

Cognitive Restructuring

I first taught cognitive restructuring to first-year medical students at SLU, and it made me realize both how powerful a technique it is and just how prevalent problematic mindsets and cognitive distortions are among young people. I was aided in the development of the presentation by Ginny Fendell, a therapist who worked with college students at Washington University in St. Louis. Cognitive restructuring is a technique that forms the basis of CBT, which, as mentioned in previous chapters, has been used by therapists for decades. If you were to see a therapist for anxiety or depression, or for maladaptive perfectionism or impostor phenomenon, chances are that they would use CBT. I have long wondered why we withhold these techniques until someone develops a full-blown mental health problem and needs to see a therapist. As one medical student said to me after a cognitive restructuring class, "I wish I had met you eight years ago, Dr. Slavin. You would have saved me a lot of suffering."

On that first day of my cognitive restructuring class, 180 students gathered in the school's auditorium during the second week of school to hear me speak, and not necessarily because they wanted to—this was one of my few classes that I had made mandatory. I welcomed them and told them that I hoped they were off to a good start. Already, they had gotten a taste of the torrent of information that they would be expected to not only absorb but master (even with the cuts in content that we had made the previous year, it was still a torrent!).

"I know that you're scheduled to have your first exam in medical school on Friday," I said, "and I'm sure there is some anxiety out there about it. I want to say a little bit about the exam. First, I'll start by stating with absolute certainty that half of you will fall below the median." Some nervous laughter rippled down from the upper rows as the students looked down at their feet or glanced at their neighbors, their eyes slightly widened in shared alarm. "For many of you," I continued, "that will be a completely new experience. Most of you have not only been above average, but you've also been at the *top* of everything you've attempted since you were three years old! I can say from my experience in talking to students in previous classes that many of you will have voices in your head if you fall below average. Voices with opinions. So, what do you think those voices will say?"

I scanned the class, looking for a raised hand. Silence. Finally, from the back right corner of the classroom, a male voice called out, "You're stupid!"

"Exactly, great, thank you!" I said, and the classroom filled with laughter. The dam had broken, and responses started to flow.

"Everyone else is smarter than you!"

"How could they have accepted you to med school? They made a terrible mistake!"

"You're going to fail this course. You'll never make it through med school."

"Yes, those are the thoughts, the voices you'll hear in your head. And there will be others too," I said. "These are the stories we are prone to telling ourselves, to believing about ourselves, and they are completely distorted and inaccurate. In many ways, they are utterly predictable. We are all susceptible, every single one of us, to problematic mindsets and cognitive distortions." I then went on to categorize each of the thoughts that they had voiced.

- "You're stupid!" (performance as identity, feeling as if I *am* this score, rather than that I *got* this score).
- "Everyone else is smarter than you!" (performance as identity and toxic comparison).
- "How could they have accepted you to med school? They made a terrible mistake!" (impostor phenomenon).
- "You're going to fail this course now. You're never going to make it through med school" (fortune-telling, magnification, and a bit of catastrophizing). (For context, the upcoming exam was one of fifty or so assessments they would undergo that semester, and *very* few students, typically 2 percent of the class or less, failed courses.)
- The thoughts as a whole (all-or-nothing thinking). Remember, I'd asked the students to imagine that they had scored *below average* on the exam, not that they had failed it! But in their minds, getting a below-average score was equivalent to failing.

Since that time, I have taught cognitive restructuring to countless groups of medical students, medical residents, hospital staff, college students, high school students, teachers, and parents. In the first part of my presentation, I define the mindsets and cognitive distortions that I shared with you, and it's fascinating to see the lightbulb moment for my students when they realize how their thoughts have held them captive, sabotaging them and causing them extreme distress—and there is such a palpable sense of relief when they understand that they are not alone in feeling this way. When I give a workshop, I have attendees complete a simple worksheet and rate the degree to which they have struggled with each of the mindsets and distortions; then I ask them to share their worksheet with one or two people next to them. What always happens next feels magical as people realize that they are not the only ones with these patterns of thinking. More than once I've heard students exclaim, "You have impostor! How could you? You're one of the most amazing people I've ever met!"

Cognitive restructuring involves three steps:

1. Notice your thoughts and feelings.

2. Label your thoughts and feelings.

3. Dispute your thoughts.

While the steps of cognitive restructuring are fairly easy to understand, they are more challenging to put into practice, for we have long-standing distorted thought patterns that need to be replaced with more accurate ones. Developing this new skill takes time and practice. Be patient with your child and yourself. No one would expect to pick up a tennis racket or a violin and play well immediately, and the same is true for cognitive restructuring. It takes practice to get better.

1. Notice Your Thoughts and Feelings

The first step of cognitive restructuring is to **notice** your thoughts and feelings. That may seem simple and obvious, but we often have so much flying at us in our daily lives that we don't slow down enough to actually perceive what we are thinking and feeling. Also, we tend to view thoughts as extensions of ourselves, rather than simply thoughts. Contemporary author and spiritual master Amit Ray wrote, "You are not your thoughts; you are the observer of your thoughts,"[7] and that is what to strive for. Noticing requires some level of mindful awareness—which involves paying attention to what's happening in the present moment. Very often we move through our day with our thoughts far away—on something that just happened, or on an upcoming work presentation, or on what to buy for dinner at the grocery store—everything except what is going on under our noses. For our teens, it's the same—they may be thinking about homework, notifications on their socials, or what to wear, attending to a thousand and one different things, without really acknowledging their thoughts and feelings.

There are a number of effective tools to cultivate mindful awareness, including breathing techniques, body scans, guided imagery, and meditation. I would never discourage these formal practices, but it can be a challenge to commit to the time and discipline required, typically at least fifteen minutes per day for meditation.[8] I prefer informal approaches to growing mindful awareness that are relatively easy to work into a daily routine and take *no* extra time to do. When I was at SLU, I used my short walk from my parking spot to my office or my office to my parking spot as a regular mindfulness practice.

The technique was simple: I focused on one of my senses, usually sight or hearing, during my two-minute walks. When I tuned in to hearing, I became aware of birds chirping or calling, the leaves rustling in the trees, the drone of traffic, and the sound of my feet striking the pavement. As thoughts appeared in my mind, threatening to pull my focus away, I noticed them and let them go without getting caught up in them, returning my attention to the sounds. Over six months to a year, I found that my mindful awareness had improved, my capacity both to focus on my senses and to attend to my thoughts and emotions in the present moment.

How to help your child notice their thoughts and feelings: When I give workshops for teens, one of the things that repeatedly stuns them is when I share that their thoughts are just thoughts—they are not facts, they are just stories, and every person has the capacity to change them. It's important for parents to share this fundamental truth with their children. It can be hard at first for kids to separate themselves from the thoughts running through their minds, but having them think about their thinking and say out loud what they are hearing in their heads can be a useful exercise: "My thoughts are telling me I need more ice cream" or "My thoughts say I'm stupid and I'm going to fail the exam." This can give kids the bit of detachment necessary to see their thoughts as just that, thoughts, and to recognize that they don't need to be attached to them or agree with them. Parents can share what their thoughts are saying too. "My thoughts told me today that I was an idiot because I locked the keys in the car and felt stupid. But it was just a thought. I let it go." Once your kids are aware of their thoughts and the way they arise in their mind, they can move to the next step.

2. Label Your Thoughts and Feelings

The next step is to **label** your thoughts and feelings. Once you've noticed a thought or feeling that you're having, especially one that is causing you distress or signaling that you are upset, it's helpful to identify if any problematic mindsets or cognitive distortions are present. Stop and ask yourself some questions:

- What thoughts are you noticing? For example, if you received a less-than-perfect job performance evaluation, or if you burned the lasagna, your thoughts might automatically turn to what a failure you are. You might be thinking, "I'm so useless" or "I'm so stupid."
- What feelings or emotions are you experiencing? Are you noticing inadequacy, embarrassment, or shame? Anxiety? Uncertainty? Perhaps anger or frustration. Don't stop with one label when it comes to your feelings. There may be many emotions involved, some hiding under others.

- What mindsets are you experiencing, and what cognitive distortions? In relation to your thoughts about your less than perfect performance review at work, you might answer, "All-or-nothing thinking." And for the burnt lasagna, you could be struggling with performance as identity.

It's important not to stop with one mindset or distortion, as it is common, as I mentioned earlier in the chapter, for more than one to come into play in any given situation. In the burnt-lasagna scenario, you might also be struggling with maladaptive perfectionism and overgeneralization.

During the process of labeling, it is vitally important to observe your relationship with yourself. The last thing you want to do is beat up on yourself and think, "There I go again, maladaptive perfectionism, I'm such a loser!" At a minimum, you want to look at your thoughts with neutrality and, ideally, muster some degree of self-compassion.

How to help your child to label their thoughts and feelings: When you first start using these techniques with your child, you will likely need to help them see and label their mindsets, distortions, and feelings. This can be done with the step of probing for understanding, not just exploring what is upsetting a child on the surface (such as an exam score or a missed shot in the basketball game), but considering the meaning and consequences that they attach to it. Perhaps they believe that they'll fail a course, be rejected by a college, or be thrown off the team. It may be helpful, as you explore the thoughts, to talk about them as the "second arrows" we discussed earlier, the harm that they can learn to control.

Initially, you might help your child to simply label their thoughts as negative or unhelpful and over time assist them in distinguishing between the different distortions and mindsets. Hopefully, with practice, your teen can begin to take more responsibility for labeling. The ultimate goal is that they will no longer need your help in this process, that they can—and will—do it independently. Once they've labeled the mindsets and distortions, they can start to address them constructively, rather than simply accepting them.

3. Dispute Your Thoughts

The final step is to **dispute** your thoughts. Often we are so used to operating through the lens of problematic mindsets or reacting according to our go-to cognitive distortions that we fail to question whether they are correct. We accept them as truth. By challenging the validity and accuracy of our thoughts we can often disrupt the cycle of negative thinking patterns. There are a number of approaches to the practice of disputing, but I have two favorites that have worked very well with my students:

- **Discrepancy:** I call the first disputing strategy "discrepancy," and it can be used with any combination of mindsets and distortions. It's a way of looking at the tone and content of the negative thoughts we direct at ourselves that makes us realize just what we're doing—and how it's harming us. It works like this. Imagine that your best friend in school comes up to you and says they got a disappointing score on an AP History quiz. Would you respond with, "Well, you're stupid. Everyone else is smarter than you. You're never going to get an A in this course. You're never going to get into a good college." Of course you wouldn't, because that would be cruel! But you might say those words, or some variation of them, to yourself. The question then is, Why would we use a voice with ourselves that we would never use with anyone else? Why be so harsh and self-critical? And what if your friend were to talk to you in this way? You'd be outraged, saying, "How dare you talk to me like that!" So, the next time you find yourself caught up in cognitive distortions or mindsets that belittle you or predict dire outcomes, or you are spinning the data about yourself in any number of unhelpful ways, you need to ask the same question of yourself, "How dare I talk to myself that way?"

- **Analyze the evidence:** The second approach is to analyze the evidence for whether the story you are telling yourself is true or false. Is it really the case that one slow split time at swim practice means you're the worst athlete on the team? And that you'll be dropped? Or if your friend doesn't respond to your texts and "leaves you on read," is it a fact that they don't care about you and don't want to be your friend?

How to help your child dispute their thoughts: When first working with your child on disputing, you may need, as with labeling, to take an active role, but hopefully with practice over time, they will be increasingly able to take the reins.

The discrepancy technique is fairly easy to utilize. If your child has thoughts or beliefs that are influenced by mindsets and distortions, you can ask them to put their words into a friend's mouth and see how they would respond to their friend. You might say, "What if Georgia came to you and said 'I'm not going back to school. I'm too stupid and everyone hates me'? What would you say to your best friend?"

You can also assist your teen in analyzing the evidence and assessing how true or untrue their narrative is by asking questions and encouraging them to do the same. If they state that they're a failure because they fell off the balance beam in a competition and they're definitely going to be dropped from the gymnastics team, you could help them think through how true that is. Is their value as a person really tied to whether they fall—or don't fall—from a piece of gym equipment? Does falling off the balance beam mean failure or is it one single error (and a common one at that) in a complex routine? Have they been successful in other endeavors? Do they know for certain that the coach will drop them?

As your teen begins to learn how to dispute their thoughts, they may find it helpful to ask themselves the following questions:

- Is this thought 100 percent true?
- Why do I think the thought is true?
- What is the evidence for this thought?

- What is the evidence against this thought?
- Am I making any assumptions?
- Am I thinking this way based on facts or feelings?

As your child becomes more practiced at disputing their thoughts, it will begin to happen naturally and they'll catch their mindsets and distortions—"Here is that pesky thought again"—and can question them immediately.

I've noticed that for some students (people in general, really), this last step of disputing is difficult to master. They may harbor a mistaken notion that beating up on themselves, letting their self-critical voice run them ragged, has been a key factor in their success. In reality, self-invalidation can contribute to rumination, anxiety, and depression, which all have potential negative impacts on a person's cognitive functioning, including attention, memory, and processing speed. When we let go of an unattainable pursuit of perfection and its many undermining effects, we increase our chances of putting in our best performance.

It is also critical to remember what the overall goal of cognitive restructuring is and isn't. It is very easy to fall into the trap of trying to eliminate your child's pain and distress. That should not be the aim. Remember, the first arrow (the event itself) will hurt and it is okay to let your child feel that pain—and to provide support by validating their feelings and being there for them. The focus of your efforts should be on the second arrow, the one that can so often compound the pain caused by the first.

Putting It All Together

Let's take a look at how cognitive restructuring works in practice by revisiting the scenario from the start of this chapter. Alex, our high school sophomore, is devastated because he got an 87 on his math quiz and is convinced this means he won't get an A in the course, his GPA will drop, he will never get into his dream school, and his life will be ruined. After Alex storms out of the kitchen, his mom waits a little while, then goes to find him. She validates his thoughts, saying that she can see why he's upset and that she empathizes with his feelings. Now that he has calmed down, she helps him notice the thoughts and feelings he was having (as teens become more familiar with the three-step process, they will be able to identify their thoughts and feelings in the moment): disappointment that he didn't get the score he wanted, upset that it meant he wouldn't get into the college he wanted, and anxiety/fear that all his plans for the future were ruined. She walks him through the various mindsets and cognitive distortions that he is experiencing and helps him to label them.

Mindsets:

- Anything less than an A leads to disappointment with himself = maladaptive perfectionism

Cognitive distortions:

- Belief that a single quiz will affect his final grade (and beyond) = magnification
- Thought that his respectable score, an 87, is a complete failure = all-or-nothing thinking
- Prediction of subsequent negative outcomes that will result from this quiz score = fortune-telling
- Jumping to worst-case scenarios that will happen because of the quiz score = catastrophizing

Next his mom, with Alex chiming in, asks questions to explore whether his thoughts are accurate and to help him create a new narrative.

"What percentage of the grade does this quiz represent?" If the quiz is only 5 percent of the final grade, it may not be true that Alex will get less than an A.

"How much does one grade in one semester contribute to an overall GPA?" Alex can use his math skills to show that getting less than an A will have a negligible impact on his GPA and that this is just his sophomore year and grades aren't as important at that point in high school.

"Do you know for sure that an 87 on this quiz will lead Carnegie Mellon to reject you?"

"Would not getting into Carnegie Mellon really mean that you couldn't work at Google? Let's research what schools employees at Google graduate from."

"Will your life really be ruined if you don't get into that school?"

"Are there other factors and/or values that are in play that can contribute to having a good life?"

As Alex comes to see that his thoughts in response to his quiz score were inaccurate and unhelpful, his mom widens the conversation further, suggesting that what you *do* in college, and how much you enjoy it, is much more important ultimately than which specific college you attend.

Practicing Cognitive Restructuring

Now that you have an understanding of the mindsets, distortions, and cognitive restructuring in action, let's put your knowledge and skills to work with some familiar scenarios. For each of the following vignettes, try to identify the mindsets and distortions at play and how you might help the teen dispute their narrative if you were their parent. If you think your child might be open to doing this with you, feel free to invite them to; but if you think they would be uninterested or resistant to it, then don't push it.

Jada's Story

Jada is a ninth grader on the girls' junior varsity basketball team. A talented athlete, she has established herself over the season as a key team member. In the last minute of a game, she commits a turnover and her team ends up losing by two points. After the game, she slumps forward on the bench, her head in her hands and draped in a towel. Several teammates stop by and offer her a hug and whisper into her ear.

Despite being the second-leading scorer for her team in the game, Jada is inconsolable on the drive home with her dad. "I lost the game for us!" she says. "I'm a terrible player. I always screw up. Everyone must hate me!" When her dad replies that everyone makes mistakes and that they all know what a good player she is, she answers, "I'm just fooling them then, I'm really not that good. Today proves it!"

1. Notice Thoughts and Feelings

The thoughts and feelings here are fairly obvious. Jada is distraught over the turnover she made. She believes the team's loss is entirely her fault and that everyone must hate her because of it. She is also frustrated with herself. To validate her daughter's thoughts and feelings, her dad can say, "It's understandable for you to be disappointed, Jada. I know this must be really hard for you because I see how hard you practice and how much you care about your teammates and how well your team does."

2. Label Thoughts and Feelings

Mindsets:

- Jada feels the need to play perfectly to be satisfied with her performance = maladaptive perfectionism
- Jada didn't say that she had made a mistake, she said "I'm a terrible player" = performance as identity
- Jada doubts her own talent as a player saying, "I'm just fooling them then, I'm really not that good" = impostor phenomenon

Cognitive distortions:

- Jada believes that her mistake makes the entire game a failure = all-or-nothing thinking
- She made just one mistake and blew this single event up into a huge issue = magnification
- She states, "I always screw up" = overgeneralization
- She focuses on the single mistake and discounts all the good things she did during the game and previous games = tunnel vision
- She is convinced that everyone is mad at her, saying "Everyone hates me" = mind reading

3. Dispute the Thoughts

Discrepancy:

- What if her teammmate had turned the ball over and believed the loss was her fault, that she is a terrible player, that she always screws up, and that everyone hates her? What would Jada say to her?

Analyze the evidence:

- "I lost the game for us!" It's a team sport, and nobody played a perfect game. Others made turnovers, but yours just happened to be near the end of the game and that's why you are focusing on it so much. If others hadn't made turnovers earlier, you would probably have had a big lead at the end of the game.
- "I'm a terrible player." Let's look at your stats for the game and for the season. One mistake doesn't make you a terrible player.

Caitlyn Clark misses more than half of her shots. No one is perfect.

- "I always screw up." Did you screw up in the last game where your team won by twenty points and you were the leading scorer?
- "Everyone must hate me!" What did your teammates say to you after the game? I saw Susie come over to console you. What did she say?

Sean's Story

Sean is a sixteen-year-old boy, early in his junior year of high school. He has recently befriended Eric, another student who transferred into his school this year. Sean suggests that they could maybe go roller skating at the local rink and Eric enthusiastically accepts. The day arrives and both have a great time, laughing, falling, and occasionally holding hands as they circle the rink. The next morning, Sean texts Eric to say how much fun he had and that they should do it again sometime. There is no response and as the day progresses, Sean gets more agitated. "Why hasn't he answered?" he asks his mom. And later, "I thought we had a great time! He must have hated it all along." "I'm never going to have a boyfriend!"

1. Notice Thoughts and Feelings

Like Jada, Sean is extremely disappointed and very upset. He is also confused and uncertain. He believes that Eric is ghosting him because he didn't enjoy his day with Sean the day before and is convinced that his lack of interest means that he will never have a boyfriend. His mother can respond, "It's understandable for you to be disappointed. I know this must be really hard for you because I know how much you enjoyed hanging out with Eric."

2. Label Thoughts and Feelings

Mindsets:

- Sean's behavior doesn't seem to correspond to any particular mindset, but his story is a good reminder that "success" pressure doesn't just apply to school and extracurriculars but can also extend to social relationships and a pressure to have boyfriends or girlfriends and to be seen as popular. The transitional path into the world of young adulthood can be fraught with concerns and fears about whether one will make it socially or not.

Cognitive distortions:

- Sean states, "I thought we had a great time! He must have hated it all along." There are numerous other reasons that could have caused Eric not to respond, but Sean has leaped to the notion that Eric's nonresponse is because he didn't have a good time or worse = mind reading

- Sean has jumped to a perceived certain future outcome based on this single event. "I'm never going to have a boyfriend!" = fortune-telling (This could also be considered catastrophizing.)

3. Dispute the Thoughts

Discrepancy:

- What if Sean's friend Jake came to him with these same thoughts and feelings? What would Sean say to him?

Analyze the evidence:

- "I thought we had a great time! He must have hated it all along." Sean's mom can recount what Sean shared after the date and that he hasn't given any evidence that Eric didn't have a good time. She can then ask about and explore other possible reasons a person might have for not responding to a text.

- "I'm never going to have a boyfriend!" Sean's mom can explore what evidence he has that this statement is true. She can counter it with the fact that he's smart, funny, and kind. And he's only sixteen years old. He has a full life ahead of him!

Cognitive restructuring is a key technique to have in your parenting toolbox—for both your teen and yourself. As you use this approach, you may be surprised by the extent to which your kid's life, your family life, and even, perhaps, your own life have been dominated by these mindsets and distortions. Many of us have unwittingly adopted, or inherited, self-deprecating ways of thinking about ourselves and our experience, and narrating those stories in ways that our kids could have picked up on. As you start spotting these patterns in your kids, working together to overcome them and reduce their undermining power, chances are that you'll begin to feel a new sense of relief, clarity, and freedom for your kids as well as for yourself.

Chapter 7

Goal Disruption Theory: Why Many Kids Crash Out When Things Don't Go Their Way

Brett is a high school senior who lives in a leafy Maryland suburb outside of Washington, D.C. When he was in the ninth grade, a good friend of his told him that he was going to a summer program at Duke and that he should try to join him. Brett convinced his parents to send him too, and he loved it there, returning for the next two summers, embracing the college atmosphere and enjoying life in the dorms. Since first setting foot on campus, he has known that Duke is the perfect school for him, and, aware of its competitive admissions, he has worked relentlessly to maintain an excellent GPA and thrown himself into a broad range of activities to burnish his résumé. He is a member of multiple clubs and interest groups, serving as president of the Chess Club and vice president of the Community Service Club, and has played on the Varsity soccer team for the past couple of years. He thought a strong SAT score was important as well and persuaded his parents to pay for a test prep course—an investment that paid off with a score in the ninety-seventh percentile.

Despite his hard work, a chronic sleep deficit, and some measure of maladaptive perfectionism, Brett has handled the stress of school fairly well, with occasional stretches of worry around exams, but no real signs of anxiety or depression. When it was time for his college applications, it felt like a no-brainer to him. He decided to apply early decision to Duke, a choice supported by his parents and his school college counselor, albeit with gentle reminders about the highly competitive process and the need to prepare applications to other schools, just in case. "Don't worry," he told his parents. "I know I'm going to get in! A plan B will just jinx my chances!"

In mid-December, Brett gets the email he's been waiting for: The admissions decision is available. He and his parents gather around his laptop at the dining room table as he logs in to the admissions portal. There's some tension in the room as he pauses for a moment. Then he clicks on the decision and his face and shoulders fall; he has been rejected. "I wasn't even deferred!" he says in astonishment. "This must be some kind of mistake! They must have sent this to the wrong student!"—and then he collapses in sobs. His parents jump in to try to comfort him. "There are a lot of other great schools, Brett. This isn't the end of the world, we can help you with applications." Brett stands up quickly, pushing back his chair. "I'm not going anywhere else," he shouts, his face contorted. "I'm going to call the admissions director!" He leaves the room, slamming the door behind him.

Caught up in a culture that sets the achievement bar high, many teens and young people—and the adults in their lives—have high-flying goals for their futures, often revolving around their academics. As competition rises and pressure mounts, it's inevitable that achieving their ambitions is not always possible, and when disaster strikes it's helpful for teens and parents to know how to handle the fallout—or better yet, to be prepared for it ahead of time. While problematic mindsets and cognitive distortions contribute significantly to kids' feelings of distress when they don't achieve what they had hoped for, they don't fully explain why some kids unravel so severely in the face of setbacks, big and small.

Social psychologist and researcher at Claremont Graduate University Dr. Jason Siegel has an answer. He calls it goal disruption theory, a "theoretical framework that outlines when an unexpected goal violation (e.g., . . . a failed exam) is most likely to cause psychological disequilibrium."[1] In my professional life, I'm fortunate to come across people with great and inquisitive minds, and Jason is one such person I met this past year. In one of our conversations, I shared my interest in adolescent mental health, and he proceeded to tell me about a theory that had helped him parent his sixteen-year-old twins. When I asked about the origin of the theory, he said that he came up with it on the basis of a number of other psychological and behavioral models that have been around for years. His answer astonished and delighted me. *No one* comes up with theories these days—most people try to prove or disprove existing ones! I told Jason about this book and asked if I could include a chapter on his theory, and he gave an immediate yes. So, with immense thanks to Jason Siegel, in the following pages I'll distill his ideas to offer a road map through the often rocky terrain of disappointments, letdowns, and failures and help you and your teen make it through to the other side.

What Happens When We Don't Achieve Our Goals?

Psychologists, neuroscientists, anthropologists, and philosophers all believe that striving for goals is a basic human drive. It has been a fundamental part of our evolutionary journey; meeting goals such as finding shelter or trapping an animal for dinner was vital to our survival and increased our chances of passing along those genes that contributed to our goal-meeting abilities. The brain also evolved to give us little hits of dopamine after achieving our objectives, helping to encourage further goal setting.

It's natural, then, that we all have goals (and hopes and dreams) in life. Goals can be big or small, personal, professional, educational, social, or related to various other aspects of our lives. They can be broad, such as a plan to eat more healthily, or specific, like climbing Mount Kilimanjaro. They can also be realistic or unrealistic. For a teen, they may involve making the freshman baseball team, getting an A in a course, receiving an invite to their new friend's birthday party, or, as in Brett's case, being accepted by a specific highly selective college. But many goals are ultimately unmet, unachieved, barely missed, dashed, or crushed. And when our goals are thwarted, we are often thrown for a loop.

According to goal disruption theory, when something gets in the way of our realizing a goal—a goal expectation violation—it can lead to disruption (a state of psychological disequilibrium), in which we become less stable in all sorts of ways. So a rejection from Duke (a goal expectation violation) can lead to emotional upset, shouting, and irrational behavior (disruption/disequilibrium). Goal expectation violations don't always cause significant disruption, and Jason's theory offers insight into when it is most likely to occur and how intense an experience it is likely to be. Given that it is somewhat predictable, we have an opportunity to better understand it, intervene when it occurs, and even, ideally, prevent it.

Everyone has experience with goal expectation violations. You might fail to get hired for a job, or you don't receive the promotion you asked and hoped for. Or you ask a person out on a date and get turned down. All of these experiences can lead to disappointment, to a change in plans, a reassessment of the future, and even some deep soul-searching. Goal expectation violations can make the world seem less predictable and less controllable than before. What had seemed so certain is now unsure, and the road ahead must be reconsidered. The violation can bring on feelings of threat and vulnerability; contribute to low self-esteem, negative emotions, and decreased motivation; and lead to psychological disequilibrium. Brett had a clear path for his future in mind, which hinged on acceptance at Duke, and now it is blocked. Imagine the feelings, distress, and disequilibrium he must feel, having pursued for years a single, narrow goal that has been abruptly dashed.

What Does Disruption/Disequilibrium Look Like?

The disruption or disequilibrium that can arise after a goal expectation violation can be manifested in a number of ways and is characterized by a measure of cognitive and emotional compromise. Brett was affected significantly. The day after his rejection, he called the admissions office at

Duke, despite his parents' advice against it, to ask if there had been a mistake, if perhaps they had confused him with another applicant. The admissions officer pulled open his file and assured him that no mistake had been made and that large numbers of highly qualified applicants were not accepted each year. At that, Brett hung up the phone, barely able to respond through his tears. He went to school in a daze, kept his head down during classes, and, sitting at lunch with his best friend, put in his earbuds and said, "I don't want to talk about it." After school, he skipped soccer practice and went straight home. There, he deflected his mom's questions, turned down his dad's offer to shoot some hoops in the yard, and disappeared into his bedroom to play videogames. When he received an email from his school college counselor offering condolences and an invitation to meet, he read it, then deleted it.

Impacts on Mood and Disposition

Failing to reach a goal or suffering a setback along the way can bring on a multitude of emotional responses as we navigate our feelings. These can include:

- A change in temperament with irritability or hostility, particularly if efforts are made to push the disappointed person back toward a balanced mood. For Brett, this immediately manifested as upset and anger when he saw that he had been rejected. Suggestions from his parents that there were still other options available to him were met with fury.
- Becoming less willing to take others' perspectives or being closed to any feedback that doesn't focus on regaining the original goal. In Brett's case, he refused to listen to advice that didn't relate to somehow getting the admissions office to reverse the decision.
- Becoming more defensive, less trusting, less willing to forgive. This development of emotional armor is a coping mechanism

that often occurs in reaction to failure, to having been vulnerable or to putting oneself "out there." It is designed to protect against similar situations arising in the future.

- Becoming more egocentric. An excessive preoccupation with one's own needs can arise as a defense mechanism as someone focuses on how much they've been affected, how terrible the situation is, and how little others can understand. In the wake of his rejection, Brett became entirely focused on himself and how his life had been ruined as a result of his rejection from Duke. He didn't consider how his behavior affected his parents but was laser-focused on his own experience.
- Feeling hopeless. These feelings can be tied to lowered self-esteem and lack of motivation as goal disruption leads people to think what's the point of even trying, of having goals at all.

Impacts on Thought Processes and Decision-Making

Disruption/disequilibrium can include a range of cognitive effects, impairing judgment and leading to rash decisions.

- Mental resources are directed entirely at understanding how the goal violation came about and fixating on achieving the original goal to the exclusion of everything else. In the days that followed his rejection, Brett could only think about how he could still get into Duke.
- Intrusive thoughts and rumination about the thwarted goal and its future consequences can increase negative emotions and decrease problem-solving skills. It's difficult to have the cognitive capacity for anything else.
- A decrease in ability to switch to other goals, caused by a continued focus on and emotional commitment to the previous goal. For Brett, this meant he had limited capability

to think about applying to other colleges, even though the deadline for regular decision applications was just a couple of weeks away.

- Less ability to come up with alternate solutions or accomplish other simultaneous goals. The focus is entirely on the goal that was violated, and how to achieve it.

Impacts on Processing and Perception

Disruption/disequilibrium can lead to changes in thought processing and perception to further impair judgment. In fact, one big takeaway that Jason Siegel taught me—and that he has used with his kids—is not to make big decisions or take drastic actions during disequilibrium as we don't have the cognitive capacity to make thoughtful choices.

- Oversensitivity, hypervigilance. In times of heightened vulnerability and stress, the body's fight-or-flight system quickly steps in to assess threat in our surroundings. This can lead to hypervigilance, a state of being on guard and keyed up that can manifest as sleep disturbances such as insomnia. In the days following his Duke rejection, Brett found it impossible to relax enough to fall asleep and spent many nights staring at his ceiling or tossing and turning until dawn.

- Exaggeration of the importance of the goal, as well as a fear of failure. When we experience goal disruption, the original goal can take on an even rosier appearance, making it all the more terrible that it is no longer possible for us, and leading to hesitation before we can be vulnerable enough to pursue another goal. Brett is not alone in viewing admission to or rejection by a dream college as akin to a life-or-death experience. Indeed, one college advising website seems to play on this high-stakes metaphor by offering an application "postmortem" (for a price) after an early decision rejection. The distress of not getting into one's dream college can be compounded by a fear of failure to get into *any* good college.

- Exaggeration of the outcomes associated with failure. The person painfully dwells on not just this specific failure but its presumed implications. Catastrophizing and fortune-telling, as described in the last chapter, run rampant.
- Tunnel vision (one of our cognitive distortions). This involves focus on the negative event to the exclusion of other positive aspects of life. Brett's hyperfocused dismay caused him to discount everything he had accomplished in high school and enormous assets such as his good health, his loving parents, and his overall prospects for the future.
- Processing that is more biased and irrational. Information perceived as irrelevant is ignored. Brett was closed to any other information or options other than appealing the rejection decision. Only when his disequilibrium began to diminish several days later could he consider listening to his parents' thoughts.
- Direct, aggressive, regressive behaviors. Teens may lash out when help or consolations are offered.
- Disregard for collateral damage as irrelevant. Those in disequilibrium can disregard the feelings of others, barking at anyone who tries to step in. Brett brushed aside the advice that calling the admissions office would likely not help and might even compromise any future interactions with them. Also, by ignoring his college counselor's email, he was not treating with care a relationship with someone whose help he would be seeking for his other applications.
- Increased commitment to one course of action. It feels like no other options are satisfactory, so a hyperfocus on this single

goal and trying to figure out how to still achieve it dominates one's thinking.

What Can a Parent Do?

Be Prepared for Disruption/Disequilibrium

As mentioned earlier, a goal expectation violation does not automatically result in disruption/disequilibrium. According to goal disruption theory, five factors can affect the degree of disequilibrium that someone might feel. As you will see, awareness of them may not be helpful if your teen is already struggling with goal disruption (more advice on that later), but it can be useful in preparing for potential negative outcomes from setbacks such as unsuccessful sports competitions or college admissions.

The nature of the violation itself. What is the event or incident that is thwarting the goal, and what is its impact? To understand this, it can be helpful to consider the following questions: How important was the goal? How close was your child to achieving the goal? Was the violation unexpected? How much effort had they put in? What are the potential consequences of not achieving the goal? It's also important to remember that the nature of the violation may appear differently to your teen than to you, and that their perception matters.

In Brett's case, his goal violation (rejection by his dream college) met many of these criteria for severe disequilibrium. His goal was extremely important to him. He not only thought that he was close to attaining the goal but was absolutely certain of the outcome before it arrived, even imagining himself moving into his dorm room and beginning his life at Duke. The violation was completely unexpected for him. He had put in years of effort to achieve this specific goal and he perceived the consequences of the goal violation as enormous (though in reality they were not). Remember that cognitive distortions, particularly magnification and catastrophizing, can make even small goal violations feel monumental.

Your child's psychological state. Are they sleep deprived? (If they are like most kids in the schools I've studied, the answer is likely to be yes.) Do they suffer from anxiety or depression? Do they have a personality disorder, a mental health condition such as borderline or narcissistic personality disorder? These conditions often involve intense emotional and behavioral patterns that can lead to stronger reactions to failure and contribute to feeling more disequilibrium. Kids with mental health disorders are more likely to struggle with the uncertainty or disappointment of goal violations and may lose their footing for a while. Engaging their therapist (or seeking one) in navigating disequilibrium is wise, especially if symptoms flare or worsen. Brett was, like many kids his age, a bit sleep deprived, which could contribute to emotional unraveling and irrational thoughts on occasion, but he didn't have anxiety, depression, or a personality disorder. His reaction, though intense, was likely to be relatively short-lived.

Personality traits. Your child's personality plays a significant role in how they respond to goal violations. Is your child generally optimistic or pessimistic? How tolerant are they of uncertainty, of ambiguity? Are they able to stay calm or to calm themselves down? What is their track record with goal violations in the past? Each of these factors can influence the degree of disequilibrium they experience. Many teens struggle with ambiguity and uncertainty, particularly those with anxiety. While those with maladaptive perfectionism may have repeatedly experienced goal violation and disequilibrium, they may not have developed skills to deal with them. Others who have learned cognitive restructuring from a therapist may have developed resilience, managing to reduce their experience of disequilibrium. You know your child best, and your sense of how they might react will be invaluable here.

Complexity of goals and identity. This factor relates to how great a part of your teen's life and/or identity the goal in question was. How many goals does your child have? Are all their eggs in one basket? For example, is their singular goal to win the high school cross-country regionals or do they play several sports? Are they hoping to gain admission to a single highly selective school or program, or have they chosen several schools where they'll be happy? Is their identity wrapped up completely in their academic performance and success? Have they always been viewed as the "smart" one? Brett checked some but not all of these boxes. He had been involved in a range of activities that he felt good about, though most of his activities had been chosen to bolster his college application. While he had done well in school, his parents had tried to avoid too heavily rewarding his academic performance, making sure he knew their love was not contingent on his success. In the past couple of years, however, his school and extracurricular achievements had narrowed to support his getting into Duke—and his rejection had stung.

The perceived availability of other paths. Does the goal violation make it feel like doors have been irrevocably closed? Was there a plan B in place, or maybe C and D? Brett was so certain of his acceptance that he neglected to do any planning for other options, in part thinking superstitiously that doing so would make his acceptance to Duke less likely. While he has plenty of other doors to open and opportunities to pursue, the one door he wanted to walk through, admission to Duke, has closed for now. It will take some time for him to get to a point where any other possibilities appear even slightly attractive.

How to Help Your Child If They Are Struggling with Disruption/Disequilibrium

If your teen has suffered a setback and is struggling emotionally, it can be difficult to witness. Our impulse is always to protect our child, to rush in and free them from pain. The first impulse of Brett's parents upon his rejection from his cherished college could have been to support what he was advocating for—to pick up the phone and call the admissions director and demand a recount of sorts. But they didn't do that. Their role—and your role—is to support the child through their distress rather than remove its cause. A first arrow has struck—the reality of the event that didn't work out—and the experience of some emotional pain is natural and expected. The following steps can be helpful to ease your teen through this process and diminish the possible effects of the second arrow:

First, try to be a calming presence (no matter what you're feeling inside). This may be a challenge as often we become invested in our teen's goals ourselves. But it's important for your emotional upset not to ignite an already-volatile situation.

Acknowledge your child's thoughts and empathize with their feelings. For Brett, this might be saying, "I know how hard you worked to get into Duke, how much you wanted to go there. It's understandable you are so upset; I know this really hurts." Initially, try to be a quiet loving presence. This is the time to stay in the moment rather than pivoting to the fact that there are lots of other great colleges out there, or that you never liked Duke in the first place. Keep your focus on validating your child's feelings.

Normalize the grieving process and the emotions and behaviors that come with it. With a big goal violation and the ensuing disequilibrium, don't rush your child too quickly to compose themselves. There is first-arrow pain that they need to feel and deal with, and you should not push to eliminate their distress. Missed goals are a loss and will need to be grieved. For Brett that meant tears and frustration, time in his room alone, and lots of videogame playing. His parents understood his need to process his emotions like this and didn't try to limit the videogames. But when he asked to stay home from school the next day, they told him no, that he'd be better off with his friends and the distraction of classes and soccer. They wanted to maintain a balance, supporting their son while keeping his routine in place. Over time, your teen should fold the disappointment into their life experience, but if you are concerned that they seem negatively affected weeks after the event, speak to their doctor or a mental health professional.

Encourage self-care. If they seem open to it, you can encourage using calming techniques in the immediate aftermath of the goal violation, such as breathing exercises if they have used them previously. They can also use calming techniques as distressed thoughts and emotions arise in the days following their disappointment. Other good self-care activities include physical activity, listening to or playing music, and spending time with friends.

Offer space if they need it (but check in regularly). Ask your child if they want to be alone to process their thoughts and feelings, and let them have some space if they need it. If they seem to be spending a lot of time alone, check in on them, especially if it's a new behavior.

Probe for understanding. Once they are more composed in the hours or days ahead, you can try to get a sense of what they're thinking. It is important to gain an understanding of what the goal violation means to them—you may be surprised that it's not what you thought. Brett didn't get into Duke, but what does the thwarting of that goal mean? Does he think that he won't have as good an experience at any other college? Does he have a future goal of being a physician and believe that Duke was the best route for that goal? Only by allowing your child to tell you—and withholding any judgments you may have—can you begin to see the situation through their lens.

Find an alternate path. As a parent, you'll have to thread the needle of acknowledging your child's distress while helping them see that they have other options available. You may have to calibrate your efforts here, not pushing too hard if they are not ready, or are completely close-minded, and/or are showing open hostility toward you. Don't rush too quickly into the development of a new plan, but once their disequilibrium has quieted and they seem ready for it, you can help them begin to develop a plan for forward movement. For Brett, that meant his parents commiserating with him and chatting with him about his disappointment a few times and then letting him be. Over the course of a week, he seemed to acclimate to this new reality of life without the prospect of Duke, letting it settle over him like a new piece of clothing. At one point as his pain lessened, his dad showed him a video by someone who had been rejected by their dream school and ultimately thrived. During the last week of school before the winter break, his mom suggested that they schedule a meeting with the school college counselor, which they did. Though Brett was quiet at first, he left the meeting resolved to apply to his second choices and maybe even to visit a couple. It felt like he was back on track.

Know your child and act accordingly. Ultimately, you know what will work best for your child in terms of timeline and how to help them shift to another path. But with constant support and understanding, and keeping their needs and well-being at the forefront, you will likely be able to help your teen as they face the inner turmoil of disappointment. Your role is to be there for them as they carry their pain, rather than to carry it for them.

Bring in a professional. Sometimes disequilibrium lingers and affects a person's ability to move forward or fully function. Fortunately, Brett was able to process his setback and find other options, but if he had remained locked in his anger and sadness about his rejection his parents would have been wise to speak with a professional—Brett's pediatrician, the school counselor, or a mental health professional—to advise them on next steps.

Getting Ahead of Disruption/Disequilibrium

You can take a number of steps as a parent to prevent, or at least lessen, severe reactions to goal violations.

Encourage the development of multiple, broader, and more achievable goals. In this way, your child is less dependent on one particular outcome and has different options to turn to if something doesn't work out. If they are determined to be valedictorian of their class, encourage them not to aim lower, but to aim wider. Help them see that a healthy pursuit of excellence in their studies—rather than chasing perfection—is more achievable. Suggest a mindset shift from outperforming others to get the one top spot to deriving satisfaction from a job well done. Encourage them to have several short- and long-term goals, large and small, in a variety of areas, so that they don't have all their eggs in one basket. Thinking outside the box of achievement culture can be good here.

If your child is set on a narrow, difficult goal, explore with them ahead of time what their chances are of achieving it. I know of a twelve-year-old who was deeply disappointed after not making the club soccer team. The reality, though, was that two hundred kids had competed for ten slots, an acceptance rate about the same as gaining admission to Harvard. Explore with them why they are so set on a particular goal. Are there reasonable and more achievable alternatives that can sit alongside their goal? Liz, a fifteen-year-old, had a goal of becoming a pediatric cardiologist. At first, her dad was proud of her ambition and was all in on supporting her goal. One day, he asked her why she was so set on this career choice, and it turned out she'd seen a TV show in which a pediatric cardiologist saved a child. As they chatted, it became clear that Liz was drawn to working in service to children in some capacity, perhaps ideally in a healthcare setting. She began to see that her goal was overly specific, that there were plenty of options available for her, and that she had years to decide on her career plans. As her dad said, "Take some time to explore what drives you, what you feel passionate about. Now's the time to try on lots of things for size!"

Encourage them or help them to develop a plan B and, if necessary, plans C and D. "It's always good to have a backup plan" is a mantra every teen should know. And it's helpful if the backup plan is an option your teen is relatively satisfied with. While Brett's parents had suggested that he come up with a plan B—which he refused to do—they could have gently revisited the topic as he submitted his application and in the days leading up to the early decision announcement. Similarly, his college counselor might have returned to the topic even after Brett refused to consider it. The reality, though, is that you can't force a child into considering a plan B if they don't want to. I recommend that any time your child sets a major goal for themselves you encourage them to work out a contingency plan—before they get overly attached to just one outcome. It's helpful to have a plan B discussion when your child is not in disequilibrium and to refer back to it if the goal is indeed violated.

Reiterate your love. Make sure your child knows that your love for them is not contingent on them meeting their goal, that you love them for who they are rather than for some specific accomplishment. Sometimes teens set their sights on a particular career, such as law or medicine, or attending a specific college, because they believe it's what their parents want. When their parent is wholeheartedly invested in their goal, the child can find it hard to back away from it even if they no longer want it—or have never wanted it.

Teach and model planfulness. Planfulness includes thinking carefully about goals, developing action plans, anticipating potential obstacles, and having mental flexibility. Higher planfulness in teens during the COVID-19 pandemic was found to be associated with lower stress, higher well-being, and lower goal disruption.[2]

Help your child try to build optimism. Psychologists used to believe that optimism was a fixed psychological trait, but research has found that it's possible to change our mindset to a more positive one, which helps us handle negative situations—including goal violations—more effectively. Ways for your teen to cultivate optimism include reframing events, writing in a gratitude journal or app each day, and spending time with people who make them happy—positive emotions can be contagious too. You can also model optimism—not an unbridled optimism but a realistic one, a faith that things will turn out okay in the long run.

Help your child develop self-efficacy and resilience by doing your best to avoid the anxiety dependence trap. Try repeatedly and consistently to get *them* to figure out how to solve problems rather than jumping in to solve them first.

Let your child get comfortable with uncertainty. When things don't go according to our best-laid plans, it's easy to feel disoriented. Developing the capacity to sit with uncertainty, to be okay with not knowing something for sure, can be an especially useful life skill. Help your child learn that there really are no certainties in life and that they can learn to handle that. You can model this yourself and talk to them about uncertainties that you've experienced in your own life. I related to my daughters how my application years ago to a prestigious master's degree program in public health was rejected. I felt initial disappointment and doubt, as the path I'd seen for myself hadn't worked out and I wasn't sure what would happen next. However, it was possibly one of the greatest professional gifts in my life as it led me to pursue my career in medical education instead. Share stories of times that things didn't work out for you. Not every story has to have a positive spin—sometimes the truth is that goal violations and the ensuing disequilibrium are painful and other options are less attractive. The point of these stories is that you found a way to get through your initial disappointment and find a different path. It's possible to build up your tolerance to uncertainty by exposing yourself to it a little at a time.

In this chapter, we've addressed important life skills that can help your child deal with and overcome the inevitable disappointments and failures that they will experience in adolescence and in their lives as adults. This is an essential element of resilience—the ability to face setbacks and ideally not just bounce back but bounce forward. A by-product of achievement culture is the sense that life is a race, a competition, and that if you don't keep "winning" along the way, your path to success will be inevitably compromised. It's no surprise, then, that many teens crash out when disappointments occur. You, as a parent, can help your child manage their goals and identities to lessen their chances of experiencing severe disequilibrium, and when goals are not met (as inevitably will happen), you can help them manage the fallout. Teaching them the tools to handle stress is an important part of helping your child navigate the demands of life, but there are also other strategies that you can use to keep them on a path to good mental health and well-being. In the next two chapters, we'll focus on working to reduce the demands and pressure they experience in school and extracurricular activities.

Chapter 8

Your Kid in School: Too Much, Too Fast—And Why Kids Feel Disengaged

Mike Nicholson, a former teacher and school superintendent in Columbus, Ohio, founded and leads Learning InspirED, a nonprofit organization that promotes student autonomy and self-directed learning in education from kindergarten through twelfth grade. Recently he developed a program for high school teachers and administrators to each shadow an individual student for an entire day so that they can get a visceral, emotional, and physical feel for a typical day in the life of a high schooler. A team at a public school in rural Ohio took him up on this opportunity, following ten middle and high school students at their own school from first to last bell. At the end of the school day Mike met with the group to debrief, and as they sat together in a circle, the principal asked the teachers for their impressions.

"It was a *long* day," said one. The others agreed. "There was a lot of sitting," said another. "A lot of material to get through, not much time before we had to move on . . . and worksheets. And so much homework assigned for each class." "Right?" added another. "I'm so glad I don't actually have to do it. I was completely exhausted by fourth period!" "And I was desperate for my phone before I even got to lunchtime." After all the teachers had shared their reflections on the day, the principal offered his own assessment: "I can't say this any other way. It sucked."

By exploring what school days look and feel like for far too many kids in the U.S. today, I hope to help you develop an appreciation for what your child may be experiencing, and for the implications this has for the kind of home life that you can strive to create. I'll start by describing the educational structures and practices that are prevalent in the U.S., how these often go against accepted educational theory and lead to poor mental health *and* poor educational outcomes, and how some schools are changing to create better learning climates. This section may feel somewhat overwhelming and even depressing, but I promise to follow with potential solutions and coping mechanisms. These will include steps you can take in your own home to create a safe space for your child, a place that reduces rather than amplifies the pressure created by school demands and achievement culture. I'll end with a focus on two contexts where you can apply your understanding of educational practices: advocating for change to benefit your child and choosing a school or a school district that will best serve their needs.

The Form and Failure of Secondary Education in the U.S.

Educational theory in the U.S. has had a long and rich history. Among its primary figures was John Dewey, a philosopher, psychologist, and educational reformer who developed his most influential theories during his tenure at the University of Chicago, between 1894 and 1904. In a series of well-regarded works[1] that continue to inform concepts of best practices today, Dewey promoted the idea that critical thinking, inquiry, and problem-solving skills form the core of a sound education—rather than rote memorization. In his book *Democracy and Education: An Introduction to the Philosophy of Education,* he states, "Were all instructors to realize that the quality of mental process, not the production of correct answers, is the measure of educative growth something hardly less than a revolution in teaching would be worked."[2] Dewey believed that learning should be student centered—that is, focused on the specific interests of each child—and should involve active engagement, including hands-on experience, rather than passive absorption of material. He advocated for curricular content to be integrated across disciplines in a way that happens in the real world, rather than separated into siloed subjects, and for courses that were designed to nurture students' moral and civic development, not simply their academics. Other progressive educational philosophies that have held sway over the years, such as the Montessori method and the Reggio Emilia approach, have followed a similar style, centering the child, proposing self-directed learning, and encouraging collaboration.

Many of these forward-thinking ideas and proposed reforms are familiar to us today—and, indeed, they ring true as they follow prevalent, commonsense notions about how we, adults as well as children, learn best. For the most part, however, though widely admired they have never been broadly implemented in American education. Currently, they are not embodied in the curricula and teaching practices of many schools across the country, which have largely opted for much less progressive modes of learning—usually in the pursuit of quantifiable ways of measuring students' proficiency through standardized courses, testing, and relentless grading systems. Improved technological tools can make learning feel modern, but frequently kids today are expected to learn in much the same way that their great-grandparents did, sitting passively at desks for much of the day and regurgitating memorized material. What is markedly different, however, is the amount of testing that goes on, the unprecedented pressure that comes with it, and, for many students, the crushing load of homework that is frequently the norm. This learning experience is a far cry from what Dewey envisioned a century and a quarter ago, and it has only gotten worse in recent years. And not surprisingly, students' well-being, including their mental health, has only declined along with it.

The teens in the schools I surveyed over the years spoke to me about the central place that school occupied in their lives, dominating their days, evenings, and weekends. It was always on their minds, always the first question out of their parents' mouths, "How was school today?" For many of them, it wasn't a place of joy and discovery; instead, it felt like a chore, something to be endured or suffered through in a battle to get somewhere else. They expressed a feeling of constant drudgery, of being caught up in the proverbial rat race, checking boxes along the way. They showed up every day and put the work in—it was all they had ever known—but the toll on their mental health was significant, and the notion of enjoying learning and the school day was strikingly and sadly lacking.

In the following pages, I explore some of the commonly seen characteristics, structures, and practices that have proliferated in secondary education (and earlier grades) in the U.S. and that parents and teens often speak to me about. Not all schools match all the descriptions below, and many of these conditions exist on a continuum rather than as a yes/no binary. However, these features are remarkably common, and as we go through them, I invite you to observe how many of them are consistent with your own child's experience of school.

Knowledge Acquisition, Memorization, and Test Prep

Many schools focus heavily on knowledge acquisition, rote memorization, and test preparation rather than deeper learning as students are taught specific content and skills that will be assessed by standardized tests. This trend has intensified in recent years and has also moved to earlier grades, in large part because of the No Child Left Behind Act signed into law by President George W. Bush in 2002 (as mentioned in chapter 5) and its 2015 update, the Every Student Succeeds Act. With a mandate to ensure that all kids, regardless of race, gender, geographic location, or socioeconomic background, have access to the same material, the acts have required that states develop academic standards and assessments and begin testing students annually, starting in elementary school and continuing into high school. By 2005–6, all states were required to test all kids in public schools in reading and math every year between third and ninth grade, and then once again in high school, and the requirements are still in place today.

These are not the only standardized tests students are required to take.

The total number of such tests administered over the course of their school years is staggering. One study of sixty-six large school districts in the U.S. found that each student was required to take an average of *112 tests* between pre-K and twelfth grade, a number that did not include optional tests, diagnostic tests for students with disabilities or English learners, or school- or teacher-developed tests.[3] A high school sophomore told me, "Sometimes it feels like all we do is prepare for and take tests; it's exhausting, and so stressful! And when we're done with one, it's on to the next one." Schools have faced substantial pressure to demonstrate that a high percentage of their students are performing at a "proficient" level so that they can receive government funding—which has led to increased pressure on teachers to "teach to the test" so that students score better.

In turn, the accumulated pressure has been passed down to students of all ages and especially high school students. These tests loom large in their lives—determining whether students graduate, what kinds of colleges they'll attend, and even future career opportunities. Kids realize the significance of these exams from an early age. One study showed that third to fifth graders experienced greater test anxiety for high-stakes standardized exams than for typical classroom testing[4]—an anxiety that flares up more often as more standardized tests become the norm until for some kids it remains at a constant simmer. Interestingly, teachers also feel more anxious about high-stakes tests. Research has shown that when teachers experience increased anxiety, stress, or pressure, they tend to teach more to the test.[5]

Passive Teaching and Learning

Not surprisingly, when test scores become a primary focus, or worse, *the* primary focus, passive teaching and learning approaches, such as relying largely on lectures by teachers, are often seen as the most efficient and effective way to transmit knowledge. Students—including the ones deemed most proficient—are the losers. There is little time for a teacher to linger over material or take a detour into related content as they must hew to a rigid content schedule. What is lost, or severely diminished, is active learning, where students are engaged in activities such as classroom discussions and debates, case-based learning, peer teaching, and group projects—proven ingredients that can inspire and energize students.

When passive teaching approaches are used, students become idle recipients rather than seekers of knowledge, and there is often no opportunity or incentive to wander from a prescribed path. Mia, a junior at a school in Providence, Rhode Island, said, "Any time we're interested in something that's not on the test, our teachers just skip over it. In the end, we stop being interested." She added that when she was younger she would try to find out more about different topics that had come up during class, usually on her own at home. But she no longer has enough free time to do that—her main focus is learning the material she's assigned so that she can get good grades.

In addition, the seven-classes-per-day schedule that students race through in the typical high school exacerbates the problem. Each short forty-five- to fifty-minute window makes it difficult for teachers to delve deeply enough to stimulate curiosity or to follow a train of inquiry down the tracks for any significant length of time before the bell cuts thinking short.

Knowledge loss—the sloughing off of acquired knowledge—is a well-documented phenomenon and is more prone to happen with curricular and content overload. If you shove enough information into a student's brain without sufficient connections, context, or meaning, students are likely to forget much of it. Ironically, then, teaching approaches that are designed to facilitate the most direct acquisition of knowledge for the purpose of standardized test performance don't even accomplish that very well. We all know what it feels like when the gears of our own curiosity are engaged and when they are not, and what effect this has on what we care about and remember.

Curricular Narrowing and Inflexibility

Educational policies at the federal and state level have led to narrowness and inflexibility in curricular content, resulting in schools that increasingly resemble a "factory" model, where every student goes through an assembly line of uniformly sequenced learning. In practice, this looks like fewer opportunities for student choice in terms of classes (less choice in electives) and little in the way of what's known as interdisciplinary content (the integration of information from disparate fields or subjects, which enables students to weave strands of knowledge into new configurations). Curiosity and creativity, so important for problem-solving and motivated learning, are too rarely nurtured beyond the younger grades and are regarded as unimportant for most kids as they advance to middle and high school. Parents and teachers are often focused on quantifiable results, hard skills that can be measured—proficiency in math and grammar, memorization of dates and scientific equations. I remember one parent who switched preschools for her child because she felt he wasn't learning anything by "messing around with water, sand, and blocks." She was delighted when he came home from his new school, reciting the names of the ships that Columbus had sailed on. This mentality, when implemented wholescale in schools for students of all ages, diminishes the creativity and joy of learning.

Surveys of U.S. classrooms that tested students on two core subjects, math and reading, found that an additional 75 to 150 minutes of weekly teaching time was added for each one—at the expense of other subjects.[6] In many schools, class time dedicated to visual and performing arts, social studies (including civics, economics, and geography), vocational classes, home economics, and physical education has been eliminated or severely diminished in favor of test prep. Students with various interests are often frustrated by the narrowed curricular focus, and those with a love for art or music often have no other options but to pursue them outside of the school day. Grace, a freshman student, related to me, "There's no room in the school day for me to learn about things I care about; the core classes just take up all of the space."

Lack of Student Autonomy

Classroom instruction is typically, often overwhelmingly, teacher directed, with limited (if any) opportunities for student-led learning or decision-making. A student in one of Mike Nicholson's surveys wrote, "Education should be self-guided, more like a library environment where the school's job is to ensure that the students have all the resources they need to learn, but how and what they actually learn is up to the individual." You can imagine how such an experience might ignite students' passion for their classes. In fact, studies have proven that when students have greater control over how and what they learn, there is a marked increase in intrinsic (or internal) motivation and higher levels of engagement, both of which can have a positive impact on learning and well-being.[7] A sweeping meta-analysis of 344 studies published in 2021 found that intrinsic motivation in students was associated with lower levels of anxiety, depression, boredom, and negative affect as well as higher general satisfaction, vitality, enjoyment, and social-emotional functioning when compared to extrinsic motivation and amotivation.[8] I'll be exploring the role of autonomy in improving motivation and mental well-being in chapter 10.

Focus on Grades, GPAs, and Awards

Recently, a teen in Ohio told me that it felt like grades were all that mattered in her life, that there wasn't room to think or care about anything else, not when she was in school and not when she was at home. The pressure of grades was always there. This continual assessment of student accomplishment is the hallmark of achievement culture, and it can contribute to the development of mental health problems and lead to a number of negative consequences, including encouraging competition rather than collaboration, incentivizing cheating, and fostering problematic mindsets such as performance as identity and maladaptive perfectionism. Ultimately, education becomes one test or one performance after another, where students are always expected to be at the top of their game. There is little room for self-expression or experimentation, and there are few opportunities for joyful creativity. The kids in the high schools that I surveyed identified their primary stressors as pressure—to score well in their exams and courses, to keep an A average, to not disappoint their parents, and to live up to their own expectations. And it seriously affected their mental well-being, taking the fun out of their daily life.

The heavy emphasis on grades, GPAs, and awards directly supports extrinsic rather than intrinsic motivation, which is characterized by internal rewards such as feeling a sense of purpose or meaning, satisfaction with oneself at overcoming a challenge, connection to others with a joint accomplishment, or simply joy in learning something new. Within that context, kids who are not committed to high achievement, or don't have the necessary support to excel, may have difficulty coming up with the motivation to study. If you have a child like this, you may feel, or worry, that there is something wrong with them; however, in many ways their behavior can be viewed as an understandable reaction and response to a teaching and learning environment that undermines their interest and motivation rather than encourages it.

Excessive Homework

As mentioned earlier, many schools follow a seven-period-per-day schedule, in which students learn in windows of forty-five to fifty minutes before moving on to the next class (or lunch). This structure tends to contribute to homework overload, especially in high-achieving schools, as the majority, if not all, of those seven classes will generate work (worksheets, reading, papers, quiz and exam preparation, and special projects) that is expected to be accomplished outside of class hours. In my studies of high schoolers, my survey asked specific questions about the time spent on homework each weekday. On average, students devoted three hours to homework—and as high as that figure is, the actual time spent, for many students, was even higher, as the average factored in students who were doing little or no homework at all.

The amount of homework varies by school, and in some schools it may be declining, but in schools that strive to be high-achieving, homework levels have likely risen in recent years, driven in part by the dramatic increase in the number of AP courses taken. Some courses, such as AP History, may carry a homework load of one to two hours per night—for a single course!—in addition to homework assigned for other classes that same day. If you add up school hours and homework, a good number of kids are putting in eleven- to twelve-hour days of academic work. Let's pause for a moment and wrap our heads around that number. Many of us have worked twelve hours per day, day after day, as adults, and we know what a grind it is and what a toll it takes. But we're not talking about adults who have chosen fields with notoriously grueling hours, or those who work multiple jobs to make ends meet; these are *kids*!

In 2006, Dr. Harris Cooper, a professor of psychology and neuroscience at Duke University, published a recommendation for appropriate homework amounts based on two meta-analyses he did that examined research on homework.[9] In formulating his guidelines, Cooper considered research on the efficacy of homework, child development, family burden, and student well-being—and one of his findings was that more than 1.5 to 2 hours a night of homework ceases to boost performance. Any time spent beyond that is likely only adding pressure, causing sleep disruption, and taking away from family time and the possibility of a kid opting to spend their time on an activity of their own choosing. His recommendation was endorsed by the National Education Association (NEA) and the National Parent Teacher Association (PTA) and has been dubbed the "ten-minute rule."[10] This simple guideline states that for each grade level, the appropriate amount of homework is no more than ten minutes a night per year of grade; in other words, a ninth grader's homework load should not exceed ninety minutes per day. This is *half* the average amount reported by teens in the high schools I studied. In countless discussions with parents, educators, and teens across the country, these higher numbers have been confirmed, making me wonder if there are any schools (at least high-achieving ones) that follow the guidelines anymore—if they ever did.

Heavy after-school academic demands can contribute to a range of problems, including late bedtimes and insufficient sleep (which I'll explore in the next chapter); significant stress; physical symptoms such as stomach problems, exhaustion, and weight gain/loss; reduced family time; decreased ability to cultivate skills outside of school; and increased family tension. The latter is often a consequence of kids struggling with or refusing to do their homework, which can set up a stressful school-parent-child dynamic. Homework can also contribute to inequities based on socioeconomic factors, as I'll explore later in the chapter.

One study of 4,317 high school students from ten high-performing U.S. high schools (four public and six private) in upper-middle-class communities found a correlation between higher quantities of homework and higher stress levels.[11] The research looked into the relationship between homework load and student well-being and engagement, as well as the ways in which homework can act as a stressor in students' lives.

On average, the students reported that they spent 3.11 hours on homework on a typical weekday (not including breaks, time spent texting, or time using their computer recreationally). Many students in the study reported experiencing stress, with 72 percent stating that they were often or always stressed over schoolwork. An astonishing 82 percent of students reported that they had experienced at least one physical symptom due to stress, with 44 percent experiencing three or more symptoms. Crucially, the data indicated "that more hours of homework was associated with an increase in school stress and physical distress." The study also noted that students who spent more time on their homework tended to be more engaged in school—but were also more stressed about their schoolwork. In addition, they were more likely to report that they experienced a greater number of stress-induced physical symptoms, had less sleep on school nights, and were less able to fit in time for friends and family. Excessive homework was compromising their ability to enjoy their lives.

Earlier, Faster

Another recent trend is to move curricular content earlier and to move through it faster. For example, algebra used to be taught in the ninth grade; now, many schools have moved it to the eighth grade, primarily so that high-achieving students can then go on to take calculus by twelfth grade and give themselves an edge in their college applications. Some observers have called kindergarten "the new first grade," as expectations for academic performance have increased significantly. Rather than question, critically, whether this tendency to accelerate the curriculum makes developmental sense for kids, serious consideration is being given to the idea of holding boys back for a year so that they start kindergarten at the age of six.

This trend of expecting more from kids at earlier ages has even trickled down to preschool. A parent of a not yet three-year-old recounted to me recently that each child in his son's class was expected to give an oral presentation each week, complete with a poster to point to. That week's topic was the Arctic. A mom of a fourth grader in Chicago told me that she spends much of her lunch break each day reviewing her son's homework assignments on the school dashboard so that she will be prepared to assist with his nightly work—because without her help it is often beyond his grasp. It's not clear why there is a push to move earlier and faster, other than a stubborn adherence to the idea that advancing quickly is always better, so why wait; however the risk is, or should be, clear. If kids are not developmentally ready for the task, then frustration, failure, and feelings of incompetence are likely to arise. Research clearly shows that students who fail algebra are less likely to graduate high school, and yet it hasn't stopped the relentless march to teaching it earlier[12]—and to what end?

Groups of Kids at Special Risk

Some kids are at particular risk for harm in the current educational structure and culture and deserve our attention. These include those with learning differences, under-resourced families, and boys.

Those with Learning Differences

I use the term *learning differences* rather than *learning disabilities*, as *learning disability* centers the problem on the kid, suggesting they're the one with the issue. But the true picture is more nuanced. Ability and disability depend to a degree on the demands placed on the individual. Your teen may have ADHD, dyslexia, or some other learning difference—but if school demands are not overwhelming, this difference may not need to lead to extra work, academic struggle, or lower grades. Learning disability diagnoses have climbed in recent years, and while some of that rise is likely due to increased awareness and detection, it may also be true that as academic pressures and demands have risen, so have the number of kids who are tested because they are struggling to keep up in an unreasonable learning environment. One student I know who has ADHD struggled in a typical seven-periods-a-day school setting but thrived in a four-class-per-day block schedule. With the traditional schedule she might, and often did, have assignments due or exams scheduled in seven classes on a single day, and keeping track of all this was a monumental task, let alone completing all the work. With block scheduling, the number of classes and accompanying assignments or exams was cut almost in half, and it was much easier for her to stay on top of her work and actually enjoy it.

Those from Less Resourced Families

As school demands ramp up, achievement pressure can magnify existing inequalities by placing an additional burden on students whose families have fewer resources. This can especially show up with excessive homework. Students from higher socioeconomic backgrounds often have easier access to homework help in the form of tutors and test prep companies. Students who have fewer resources at home, whose parent(s) work or are absent from home for long hours, whose parent(s) have had less formal education, who have limited access to computers or technology, who have a role as a caregiver, or who have an after-school job are greatly disadvantaged when it comes to dealing with larger homework loads.

Boys

There is growing research evidence and concern that our educational system is not working for boys. While high school dropout rates have fallen in recent years, the rate for boys is almost 50 percent higher than for girls, 6.3 percent versus 4.3 percent.[13] Boys are more than twice as likely as girls to be suspended or expelled from school.[14] Not surprisingly, the gender gap in college enrollment is substantial and growing. Fifty-seven percent of college students and 61 percent of graduate students are now female.[15]

The Overall Impact on Kids' Mental Health and Well-Being

When these various aspects of a typical school experience are added together, the negative impact on students' well-being can be substantial. Their long hours spent on schoolwork both inside and outside of classrooms and the heavy burden of stress it places on them have become accepted as necessary if they are to succeed in a competitive climate. The idea that school might be inspiring, or interesting, or even equipping students to collaborate across difference in an ever-polarized world almost seems long-forgotten, abandoned along the way.

The narrow focus on simple knowledge acquisition gained through passive learning and testing has resulted in many kids who are, understandably, stressed, uninterested, and disengaged from learning. It may seem obvious that frequent testing, competition, and academic demands contribute to anxiety and depression in students, but we need to pay attention to boredom too. There is evidence that it is on the rise in schools—occurring in both low- and high-achieving students.[16] A 2020 study of U.S. eighth, tenth, and twelfth graders found a significant increase in boredom, with students reporting a nearly 2 percent increase every year from 2008 to 2017.[17] We need to be mindful of the potential negative impact of boredom and disengagement on mental health and well-being. Studies have consistently shown associations with depression, anxiety, substance use, decreased quality of life, and risk-taking behaviors.[18]

Innovations in Schools

The outlook may seem bleak in U.S. education, yet some schools and teachers have tried to bring changes to the school day in an effort to make learning more appealing and less stressful, to accommodate students' interests, to foster their curiosity and joy, and to bolster their well-being. The shadowing experience in the public school in Ohio described at the beginning of this chapter galvanized the start of a change movement with a reduction in the number of class periods per day, an expansion of electives, and the development of a "Flex Friday." In this program, eleventh and twelfth graders can pursue a personal interest through shadowing experiences or internships outside of school, often with local organizations and businesses. The school is also making efforts to increase active, student-centered learning within the core curriculum.

One of the most common changes in schools to improve student learning, engagement, and well-being is to move to block schedules with four periods per day rather than the typical seven. Other schools are finding ways to offer more flexible schedules so that students can follow their passions *in* school, rather than out of school. Many performing arts schools, often public magnet schools, confine their core academic classes to the morning to free up time for students to pursue their artistic interest in the afternoon—their academic achievement appears not to be compromised.

Village High School, a public school in Colorado Springs, has moved all of their core curricular content to an online platform, freeing up time for transformational teaching and learning that focuses on what kids have a passion for learning, and allowing significant time for electives or pursuing outside interests, with support from teachers as needed and desired. Deadlines are set for the whole course rather than for individual assignments. Mentorship is also key, with each student able to choose their own mentor, who becomes their trusted adult—someone looking out for them, advocating for them, and helping them navigate challenges. The outcomes have been superb, with students and teachers reporting high levels of engagement and student autonomy. To answer an obvious question of how this shift has affected student performance on standardized tests, there is no evidence that it has suffered at all. Another school, High Tech High in San Diego, has led the way in project-based learning in which teaching and learning are centered on students' active engagement in collaborative projects with their peers and teachers.

Despite the pressures to teach to the test and meet state-mandated standards for content to be covered, some teachers are shifting to a different way of running their classes, allowing their students much more freedom, often informed by changes they had to make during the COVID pandemic. Andrea Vescelius teaches AP Language and Composition in the Columbus, Ohio, suburbs. She has moved from a teacher-centered approach to one that gives students much more autonomy in what and how they learn. One example is Designed Ingenuity, a framework they engage in three times per year in collaboration with Catalyst Learning Labs, a nonprofit organization that helps teachers and school leaders unleash student engagement. Students choose a project and follow their own curiosity to learn, gain personal insight, and create new meaning for themselves. Topics for the projects are wide-ranging and have included dreams, social justice, outer space, gambling, AI, and specific stocks in the stock market. Students conduct their own research, create connections, and then produce a creative artifact of their own choosing. Examples include a video with voiceover, an album cover, an app, and in one case a calligraphy scroll in Chinese characters by a student who was inspired to start learning Chinese. Andrea's students describe feelings of profound joy in learning, an "oasis" from the typically stultifying academic experiences in many of their other classes.

While some schools and teachers are embracing and enacting much-needed change, far too many remain stuck, continuing to focus on passive styles of teaching and learning that align with state standards and test performance rather than offering students an education that promotes engaged and joyous learning. The reality is that many schools are not likely to change, especially without parental involvement, and in the Supplemental Resources at the end of this book, I'll provide ideas for getting involved in advocacy campaigns to bring about changes in your own child's school.

What Can a Parent Do?

Mitigating the Harms of Schools at Home

When your teen comes home after school, they may be overwhelmed by the long day and the enormous amounts of schoolwork they need to do.

They may feel a sense of pointlessness to the relentless grind of their lives—but since they don't have time to reflect, they just keep going, trying to maintain high scores to keep their grades up. Some kids may be disengaged or feel hopeless, lost in a system that doesn't work for them. It may seem to you as if much of what goes on in their schools is out of your control—and some of it is—but there are still a number of really important ways in which you can mitigate the harms and support your child.

Create a low-pressure zone: Given the demands of the typical school day, it's essential that parents strive to create a home life that doesn't add to the burden that teens are already shouldering but rather aims to lighten their load and protect them from further harm. You want your home to be a place of refuge, as much as you can make it one, from the nonstop pressure they may be feeling.

I'm not talking about setting up a spa-like atmosphere for your child or swaddling them in bubble wrap. Instead, I'm suggesting that you acknowledge to yourself and to them that they have a lot on their plate and that you're not going to pile on with constant nagging about homework or questions about grades or their GPA. Allow your home to be a place where your teen is a student as well as a member of the family with other identities—someone who can hang out with friends, or goof around with siblings, watch bad TV, make popcorn, take out the trash. Try to create a place where they can be themselves, where they don't have to be constantly on, or achieving, or perfect. Encourage them to be their whole selves, even when it means falling apart at times, processing difficult feelings, and registering out loud the ups and downs of daily life. Let them know that they can rest in the assurance that they won't be judged and that they can always count on your love and support.

There's a common behavior known as "Stanford Duck," a term coined by Stanford undergraduates, but the phenomenon it describes is found in other colleges as well (at Penn, for example, it is known as "Penn Face"). It refers to the idea of students presenting an image to the world of effortless success, like a duck gliding across a lake, so peaceful, so calm. But if you look under the surface, the duck's feet are paddling hard—just like students who are trying to stay afloat but hiding their struggles. This behavior isn't just limited to college students, for high school students tell me that it is widespread in their environment as well. I believe it is essential to kids' mental health that they have a space in their lives where they don't have to pretend to be perfect or to have everything under control. You can let your teen know that they don't have to be a Stanford Duck at home, even if that's the image they want to portray at school. Try your best to create a home environment in which they feel safe revealing their furious paddling to you.

One way to do this is to check in with them regularly to hear how they are doing, resisting the urge to minimize or contradict what they share. If they're struggling, offer an unqualified acknowledgment, along with simple words of reassurance such as "This must be so hard, I'm sorry that things are so difficult."

Some parents may read this section and think that I'm suggesting you handle your child with kid gloves because they're going through a lot. I'm not. I believe they still need discipline, routines, and responsibilities at home. What they don't need is to receive additional pressure from you or to feel that they can't be open about their feelings at home.

Be more of their parent, less of their academic coach: Your role is to parent your whole child in all their complexity rather than focusing too heavily on one aspect of them, such as their academics or their college aspirations. This can be a difficult balancing act given the culture we live in. You'll want to show interest and support while allowing them to take primary responsibility for their schoolwork and their college applications. Ideally, this should begin in earlier grades so that by high school you are not overinvolved in your kid's homework; however, it's never too late to start. Try to consistently encourage your child to speak with their teacher if they are having a problem with mastering course material or managing their homework, rather than jumping in too quickly to assist them. Stating that it's normal to not know all the answers all the time can go a long way toward alleviating worry. Given the high demands at many schools, you may at times need to offer your help to keep your child afloat. Remember, though, that in general, your role as your child moves through high school is to help them transition to adulthood by encouraging independence while offering wholehearted support. Your role is not to badger them into getting homework done or to help them maintain a perfect GPA.

Show unconditional love and prioritize emotional connection: Suniya Luthar's research has consistently shown that emotional connection with parents is a vitally important protective factor for child and adolescent mental health in the face of achievement pressures at school and in the community.[19] Knowing, or accepting, that your relationship with your child is key to their well-being, do what you can to make time and space for an undistracted connection with them. For one thing, avoid overemphasizing outcomes and (inadvertently) communicating that your love is contingent on your child's success. Practice authentic listening. In other words, focus on thoroughly understanding what your child is feeling and experiencing, rather than jumping into a problem-solving mode (this may be harder than it sounds, especially if you are expert at the latter). Take the time to sound them out. *How are you really feeling?* Sometimes they may just want to be heard.

Step up and speak out: As a parent, you know best how your child is doing—especially if you have encouraged them to let their guard down and be their true self at home—and you have a good feel for what and how much they can realistically handle. If they announce over dinner that they're planning on taking seven APs, it's okay for you to ask them about it rather than automatically accepting their decision. In a culture that says more is always better, you may have to be the level-headed adult in the room who says "Enough!"

I believe that it is appropriate to firmly intervene in other situations, bedtime being one. It might be reasonable to occasionally allow your child to stay up late to do homework, but at times you need to put your foot down and insist that they close their books and turn off their computer. Limits may also need to be imposed. If your teen wants to apply to twenty colleges because their closest friend has, it is appropriate to simply say no, that's too many (and provide a good rationale). Other examples where limits may be needed include planning to apply only to Ivies, joining an excessive number of interest groups/clubs, or not eating dinner in order to study. I find that parents are often caught in the middle, not wanting to get in the way of their teen's success or discourage their ambition but feeling in their gut that something is off. It's okay to trust your instincts and put your teen's well-being—and your sanity—first.

Take a self-assessment check: It's easy to get caught up in achievement culture, and sometimes we are so immersed in it, or it has become so normalized, that we don't realize that we are. It can be helpful to ask yourself some questions and reel yourself back, if necessary.

- Are you overly invested in your high schooler's academic accomplishments?
- Do you feel that your child's achievements at school reflect your parenting?
- Are you adding your own stress around standardized testing?
- What do you usually talk about with your teen? Is the primary focus school and grades?
- When was the last time you discussed your values with your child, if ever?
- Do you ask your child about test results or grades as soon as, or soon after, they get home from school?
- Do you check the school portal? If so, how often?
- Have you set your sights on an elite college for your child?
- Do you believe that their enrollment in an Ivy League (or equivalent) college will ensure their future success and happiness?

The idea here is to help yourself take a step back and question the narrative that we have all been sold: that getting into an elite college is the gateway to success. A number of outstanding books like *Where You Go Is Not Who You'll Be,* by Frank Bruni, and *Excellent Sheep,* by William

Deresiewicz, have debunked the myth that attending a highly selective college provides substantial advantages in finding success and happiness.[20] In his book *David and Goliath,* Malcolm Gladwell made a case for the potential advantage of going to a less elite college in a chapter on being a big fish in a little pond.[21] Ultimately, it can be a good idea to reflect on your own role in applying pressure on your child and whether it is beneficial to them, to you, or to your family.

Making a Pact About the College Applications Process

Many parents find themselves enmeshed in the web of the college applications process, even if they vowed they would stay out of it. In some ways, it can be a challenge not to be involved as it is often such an intensive, all-encompassing experience with many moving parts playing out for the greater part of a year or more. Frequently, parents travel to visit colleges with their teens, falling in love with some of them along the way, even while finding it hard to imagine that their child might be living there, away from home, all too soon. One teen told me, "It was so embarrassing. My mom asked *all these questions* at one of the information sessions—it was as if she was applying to the college herself!"

A lot of parents put pressure on their teens both about where to go to college as well as during the application process. Some want their child to attend the same school that they went to, while others are rewriting college essays and emailing the college counselor. Before you get involved with your teen's applications, it can be helpful to take a step back and acknowledge that this is a stressful time for teens and parents. You may all view the stakes as high—but remember that they are only as high as you allow them to be. Promise yourself that you'll try your best not to add more pressure to an already anxiety-inducing situation. To this end, you may find it useful to make a pact with yourself (or with your teen, if you prefer) to help you navigate the process. Some schools use a family and school pact that centers the teen's well-being, such as one offered through the Making Caring Common Project at the Harvard Graduate School of Education.[22] I've compiled my own, inspired by my conversations with parents and teens, and I invite you to use it and modify it as best works for you and your family:

A Sample Pact:

- I will remember that this is my teen's journey and try to allow them to lead the conversation.
- I will listen to what my teen is hoping for in a college experience and support that, rather than jumping in with what I think would be good for them.
- I will work on playing a supportive role while allowing my teen to lead. If during the process, my teen asks me to be involved in a different way, we can reassess.
- I will help my teen consider a variety of schools, allowing them to see what feels like a good fit for them.
- I will not judge or rank colleges or disparage my teen's choices. I will not share my preferences unless asked for my input—and even then I'll keep my teen front and center in my thought process rather than my own needs and aspirations.
- I will encourage my teen to handle the process themselves—including making appointments with colleges, arranging meetings with the college counselor, signing up for tests, asking for references, and filling out online applications.
- I will not become overly attached to a single outcome.
- I will not allow the college search to dominate our lives, but will focus on other aspects of my teen's life as well—such as their friends and interests.
- I will collaborate with my teen's school college counselor.

Some days you may find that you've been overly involved, nagging your teen to get their college essay done or asking them—again—if they've scheduled appointments or emailed an admissions counselor. Instead of worrying that you've broken your pact, you can give yourself grace, take a deep breath, and take a step back. Researcher Suniya Luthar's quote may be useful to bear in mind: "As I often tell young people, including my own children when they were applying to college, you'll get an education. It's alright. You'll get an education. Life does not begin and end at being at the top."[23]

Advocating for Your Child

As a parent, it's important to do your part at home in supporting your child's mental health, but, as I've shown, schools have an enormous impact on their students' well-being and should assume some responsibility too. In the Supplemental Resources at the end of the book, I offer material for bringing change to schools and helping parents develop an advocacy campaign to get education systems to put our kids' mental health first—and I encourage you to take a look. Here, however, I provide suggestions to help you advocate for your own child at school and advice on dealing with common circumstances such as a teacher who is giving excessive homework.

In my experience, despite stories of dreaded helicopter and snowplow parents, many parents are hesitant to reach out to school administration to express concern or lodge a complaint when their child is encountering a problem. They may be facing unwarranted amounts of homework or a teacher who is moving too quickly through a topic or covering an inordinate amount of material in a class. Often parents don't want their advocacy to reflect negatively on their child (getting them labeled the troublemaker's child) or give the impression that their child is struggling academically; consequently, they often stay silent.

In one case relayed to me by a parent, a teacher assigned a new Shakespeare play (and an accompanying paper on it) each week for an entire semester. In another, a teacher regularly assigned two or more hours of government and politics homework each night, much of it busywork, while a biology teacher taught her eleventh graders from a college textbook. To my mind, none of those practices are reasonable, and parents would be well advised to say something, as they can see the negative impacts on their kids. It is not unusual for the teachers involved to be senior staff members who are held in high esteem for their commitment to academic rigor and student learning, making them more immune to complaints and resistant to change.

Here is a succession of steps you can take to intervene:

- Check in with other parents to see if they share your concern. It can be hard to take the first step and reach out, but very often you'll find that your misgivings are shared.
- If your concern relates to homework, check if there is a homework policy in place, and if the teacher is flagrantly disregarding it, share your concern with school administration.
- If no such policy exists, meeting with the teacher one-on-one is a good next step. It is best to have specifics regarding your concern (such as homework assigned and hours being spent) and an outcome in mind. Keep the meeting friendly and collaborative. If, however, your discussion doesn't yield satisfactory results, then bringing the issue (along with your allies' support, if possible) to the attention of the administration is a good next step.

For further advice, I recommend that you peruse the Supplemental Resources at the end of the book.

Choosing a School or a District

Some of you may be able to choose a high school or school district, and if so, you are fortunate, as many in the U.S. do not have the privilege of exercising the choice, even when some school choice exists. If you are able to choose, it's crucial to make sure that rigorous academics are not the only criterion on your list. Many parents have shared with me that they moved to a particular community primarily because of the high rankings of the public schools, or private schools, in *U.S. News & World Report*—specifically with regard to their excellent test scores and proven track record of admissions to highly selective colleges. It's understandable that parents pay close attention to these factors; however, caution is warranted. If you're choosing a school, or school district, solely on this basis, you may find, or your child may find, that the achievement pressure and stressful environment are part and parcel of the school you choose.

Here are ways of discerning—in advance—the difference between a strong academic focus (which there is nothing wrong with) and a culture of relentless pressure that can contribute to anxiety and depression in teens.

If a school seems overly focused on course loads, APs, and college acceptance rates, and repeatedly brags about the "rigor" of their academic program and its reputation for success in getting students into Ivy League schools or other elite colleges, it could be a red flag. Unless there is a marked difference from the structures and cultures described earlier in the chapter and/or objective evidence to the contrary, this laser-sharp focus may crowd out other aspects of the student experience and contribute to poor mental health of the student body. If down the line you were to challenge the excessive assigning of homework, or theater rehearsals that stretch into the night, or a superintensive practice schedule for sports, you might meet with an answer like the one Emma's parents received—that many parents are asking for more, not less.

Ultimately you need to ask yourself, What do you want for your child? What does your child want? Are you willing to risk your child's mental health in pursuit of acceptance to an elite college—that may not be a better path to "success" and financial security? Does the school understand—and embody—that "well rounded" does not mean relentless pressure on every front? Do they place limits on the number of AP classes students can take at a time? Do they take pride in their ability to offer their students opportunities to pursue their own interests? Is there substantial elective time? Do they have a strong arts program? Do they embrace active teaching and learning approaches such as project-based and/or problem-based learning? Do they nurture curiosity and empathy?

Be prepared to ask questions about how seriously schools take their students' mental health. Are they proactive, preventive, and protective? Or do they take more of a Band-Aid approach, connecting students with anxiety, depression, and other mental health conditions to mental health resources, often beyond the school? A word of caution, though, if your child applies to high-achieving private schools. You may want to be careful about asking these questions of school administration, as it could jeopardize your child's chance of entrance to that school if it does turn out to be a good fit. Administrators may not take kindly to these types of questions as they don't want parents who are going to be potential "troublemakers." To get information about the school's practices, it may be safer to talk to parents whose kids are already enrolled in the school.

Daring to Do Something Different

Some parents (and teens) are opting out and choosing a different path—and this may be right for you as well. A SLU medical graduate who is the mom of a toddler is excited to have her child attend the local public schools in the mixed-income neighborhood where she loves living, rather than to relocate to a community with more highly rated public schools or chase admission at one of the elite private schools. She believes that achievement pressure and academic demands are likely to be elevated in the other schools and doesn't want her daughter's mental health to be compromised. She also values community and the benefits of having her child develop friendships with kids and families who live nearby. Recently, an eighth-grade student toured several private schools in the San Francisco Bay Area, all with impressive track records for college admissions. After consideration, the student told her mom that she preferred the local public school, saying that at the private schools the students and the parents seemed "too intense." Surprised, her mom replied, with some doubts and concerns in her mind, "Are you sure?" "Yes," said her daughter, so the mom moved to acceptance and they decided to go that route.

The mom told me of the pressure she felt as a parent to opt for one of the schools that seemed to promise success and said that her daughter's decision to attend her preferred school had caused her to question herself.

Was she doing the responsible thing as a parent? What would other people say? Should she have insisted that her daughter try private school for a year and see? Ultimately, though, she realized it was okay to "lean out," as she put it. And that's a wonderful message that I want you to embrace if it feels right. Leaning out doesn't make you any less of a committed, caring parent. Rather, it may be the wisest choice you could make given the negative impacts that achievement pressure at so many high-achieving schools is having on our kids.

Kurt and Jennifer have consistently leaned out since their son, Peter, was young. Kurt grew up in western Europe and was mystified by the achievement culture he saw when he moved to the U.S. and began work as a minister at an elite college. There, he saw the impact of a pressure-cooker system on those who were the "winners" in the college admissions race—depressed and anxious students who were often fragile in the face of what seemed like relatively small threats to their well-being, such as not being accepted to an exclusive student club or having plans for a summer internship fall apart. Kurt no longer works at the college, but the memories of the students' mental health struggles have remained with him.

Jennifer, for her part, grew up in a high-pressure educational system and knows the negatives firsthand. Their experiences affect the way that they parent their son. They elected to send Peter, who is now in fifth grade, to the local elementary school in their mixed-income community, where he is thriving. His homework load is manageable, and he has time for free play with his friends and for family dinners and activities. Kurt and Jennifer opted to refuse acceptance for Peter to the advanced academic track, much to the surprise of the school, whose staff often see parents petitioning and pressuring for the opposite outcome. But they were insistent—they did not want school to be a high-pressure zone. Peter is relatively early in his educational journey, and next year he will move on to the local junior high school. His parents see no reason to change course for him.

Julia, a young woman who went to high school in that same district, has also thrived. She was enrolled in a private middle school but was frustrated by its small size and pressed her parents to allow her to transfer to a public high school. The parents agreed and she flourished there. She was challenged by her coursework, but homework loads were manageable overall (except for one notorious history teacher), allowing Julia the time to see friends outside school and, as she says, "to have a life." Even when she didn't enjoy all of her classes, she had her friends, and school didn't take up all the space, so she could find enjoyment elsewhere. Achievement pressure was muted and Julia sailed through without experiencing depression or anxiety. Her academic future wasn't compromised, as she gained admission to her top choice—a large, highly selective university in the Northeast. Her mother believes that Julia was likely better served in the college pursuit than if she had attended a prestigious private school. But she also added that if Julia hadn't gotten into her first choice, she would have been happy at many other colleges on her list. Her goals for herself didn't begin and end with one elite college.

As you and your teen navigate the pressures of the school system, I hope this chapter has helped you feel more empowered to take matters into your own hands to push back against societal messages of the need for constant achievement. Listen to your inner voice and let it guide you as you shift your mindset and extricate yourselves from the success trap. In the next chapter, we'll extend this practice to after-school and extracurricular activities, which are likely taking over your evenings, weekends, and holidays. Take a moment to breathe deeply before you dig in.

Chapter 9

Your Kid After School: The Overcommitment Trap

"You want to know what's ridiculous?" exclaimed Daniela at a recent end-of-summer potluck. "We haven't been able to go camping *even once* this summer with the kids! Every weekend is filled with soccer tournaments and can't-miss practices. And what's worse, we did this to ourselves—we're the ones who signed them up! And then, once they'd signed up, we didn't want to let them skip. We've already paid the fee and they've made the commitment, and we need to teach them to honor it. But we are clearly doing something very wrong if we can't spend even one weekend relaxing together."

Does this scenario sound familiar? Maybe it's swim meets or hockey games or play rehearsals that get in the way of family time for you. The potluck in question was held for seven families—but two had to cancel at the last minute because of unforeseen scheduling conflicts, and of the five that did attend, the parents were coming and going throughout the afternoon, taking this kid here and picking that kid up from there. Daniela was bemoaning the loss of a weekend getaway, but really, these families were struggling to find even a single night of unscheduled time.

It's not just school that is a relentless, frenzied pursuit of success. Life beyond the last bell has become equally harried as kids throw themselves into sports, the performing arts, after-school clubs, extra courses, college prep, and tutoring—with their parents serving as chauffeurs, snack providers, backstage volunteers, and supporters-in-chief. While some of these activities stem from genuine interest, increasingly they are the consequence of parental and teen anxiety related to competitive college admissions and an ever-escalating arms race to see who can do the most or be the best. Many schools play into this competitive trap too, lengthening and intensifying sports practices while their theater and dance productions seem to have grown ever more expansive in ambition and time commitment. In many cases, these activities are rewarding for kids and can provide opportunities for growth, self-discovery, and joy. However, when they become too time consuming, and especially, as we will explore later in the chapter, when they are overly pressured, accompanied by high expectations from adults, and competitive, they can come at a serious cost to mental health. Fortunately, there are solutions for parents and kids trapped in an extracurricular hell, and I'll chart a path forward for how we need to—*and can!*—change this dynamic.

In the last chapter, I described how extensive homework is for many teens, eating into their evenings and nights, and yet it is just a portion of their after-school responsibilities. In my high school studies, kids reported an average of five hours per weekday spent on a combination of homework and extracurricular activities like sports, drama, band, and clubs. These activities exact a huge time commitment, at times with intense psychological pressure and often, in the case of sports, strenuous physical demands. Yet rarely are they questioned as potentially detrimental to our teens' mental health, or if they are, rarely are actions taken to rectify the situation.

The Trap of Varsity and Club Sports

More than eight million students participated in U.S. high school sports in the 2023–24 school year, a record number according to the National Federation of State High School Associations.[1] In general, teens in varsity athletics practice two hours every school day, though it can be longer. Some sports have an even greater time commitment. Swimming programs typically hold afternoon practices five days a week, lasting up to two and a half hours—and it is common to also have morning practices several days a week that start as early as 5:30 to 6:00 a.m.! Meets and games for high school sports often stretch into the evening and can take place away from school—which means a team bus ride back to school before students can even start to head home. A typical afternoon and evening for Brittney, a high school basketball player participating in an away game across town, involves taking a thirty-minute bus ride with her team, watching the junior varsity game, warming up, then playing her game, quickly changing, taking the bus back to school, riding home with her dad, and finally walking in the door exhausted at 9:30 or 10:00 p.m. Instead of being able to shower, have something to eat, relax, and get some sleep, she still has homework to do. For athletes like Brittney, if it is a heavy homework day or the night before a big exam, taking time for dinner or checking in with family members may be an impossibility. It's likely that after arriving home late, they'll be up and studying past midnight, long after the rest of the house has gone to sleep.

It's not just a problem for varsity-level kids, though: 54.6 percent of kids ages six to seventeen participate in organized sports in what is now a $40 billion-a-year industry—twice that of the National Football League.[2] Many of these kids are in "club" sports—competitive athletic programs outside of school systems that are talent based and that kids must try out for. They involve practices, games, tournaments, and often travel (sometimes across states), and they are frequently imbued with a highly competitive culture. Parents have varying reasons for enrolling their kids in these sports, including skill development, exposure to competition, social interactions, and promotion of discipline. For older athletes, there is the chance to play at a much higher level, experience more intense competition, and showcase their skills in front of college recruiters, increasing their chances of gaining admission to an elite college and/or receiving a college scholarship. Many parents have told me that participation is so widespread in their communities that they worry that their child will have no one to play with, or nothing to do, if they aren't enrolled.

Some club sports, such as soccer, hockey, and gymnastics, start as early as six years of age, with travel teams starting by age eight. One dad recently recounted to me that a fellow parent had asked if he had a baseball coach for his six-year-old. When he said no, the other parent replied with genuine concern, "He'll never make the club team, then." As children grow older the intensity continues and the time commitment increases. Olivia, the eight-year-old with maladaptive perfectionism (whom you met in chapter 1), was involved in club soccer with practice twice a week and games on the weekend. Her older brother also played on a club soccer team, with three nights of practice and weekend games. Each evening one of their parents would drive them to an outer suburb, some twenty-five minutes away, for practice from 5:00 to 7:00 p.m. Three nights a week, Olivia attended her brother's practice sessions and two nights a week he went to hers. By the time they made it home, they were hungry and exhausted. They are not the only ones. Many families have shared stories of evenings and weekends spent ferrying different kids to practice and games all over town and beyond. What is lost in all of this frenzied activity is quality family time and free play, and the latter, it turns out, is vitally important for child development, as I'll explore later in this chapter.

By the time athletes are in their teens, they are often encouraged to focus intensely on a single sport so they can be as competitive as possible. One mom told me recently about her thirteen-year-old son Jordan, who was a pitcher in club baseball. An overzealous coach, eager for success, pressured him to play so much that Jordan eventually needed Tommy John surgery to repair a torn ligament in his elbow, a surgical procedure that was historically needed only in professional baseball players. In recent years, however, the majority of these procedures are being performed on teenagers. Researchers found that fifteen- to nineteen-year-olds account for the highest percentage of Tommy John surgeries (56.8 percent) and that the rate is increasing by 9.12 percent a year.[3] With the need to excel and stand out from the crowd, many teens are playing competitive baseball

all year round in high school and club leagues. There is little time for their bodies to rest and recover.

In addition to the time, energy, and physical costs associated with club sports, there are significant financial costs. According to the latest Aspen Institute Project Play parent survey, in partnership with Utah State University and Louisiana Tech University, the average amount that parents paid for one child to participate in their primary sport rose 46 percent between 2019 and 2024. Expenses can easily reach $1,000 per child per year, and if your child is on a travel team, has a private coach, and/or is in a sport with expensive equipment costs (like hockey), they can mount to $5,000 to $10,000 per year or more.

Many teens choose to continue with club sports when they enter high school, often because they have reached an elevated skill level that they want to maintain. Some decide to forgo varsity sports completely, while others take part in both. Participation in club sports at the high school level often entails a year-round commitment, higher intensity, greater achievement and time pressure, and regional, national, and even international travel.

Kristin, a sixteen-year-old ice hockey player in Minnesota, played in the winter season on her high school team and then continued to play the remainder of the year on a club team. She loved the sport, the thrill of winning, and the camaraderie of her teammates, but she had paid a big price for her involvement. The year-round commitment on top of schoolwork had left her feeling fatigued and burned out, as she had no real downtime at all. During the winter season, she had struggled with injuries including a shoulder sprain, a fractured collarbone, and chronic wrist pain, and in the last two years she had suffered three concussions. The most recent concussion had caused nausea and headaches while reading and had led to her missing a month of school as well as her SATs. Now she felt behind on her courses and college prep and faced a mountain of catch-up work—it was overwhelming. Her parents were drained as well, both physically and financially, though they tried not to show it. They devoted enormous amounts of time shuttling her to practices and traveling with her to out-of-state tournaments, and had sacrificed in many other ways, such as not going on a family vacation in more than three years. They had been hoping that Kristin would get a hockey scholarship, a long shot at the best of times, but with her recent injuries it seemed even less likely. Despite the significant costs, Kristin still loved the sport—imagine what it would be like if she didn't!

Club sports can become a dangerous trap. For many families, participation may begin innocuously enough—you might enroll your child in a sport because they show an interest, or perhaps all their friends have joined and it seems like it will be fun for them. As the years go by, practices and commitments ramp up and competitions become more intense. You may start to have doubts about the wisdom of spending so many resources in this way, but many parents and kids have conveyed to me that once they're on this train, it's simply too hard to step off. One parent told me of the night he and his wife were driving their daughter through heavy rain from Boston to New Jersey for a volleyball tournament, and he turned to his wife and asked, "What the hell are we doing?" A great question! And yet they continued to support their daughter's involvement in the sport after this epiphany.

For some families, their child's athletic talent may appear to be a pathway to a college scholarship one day. For others, it's a shiny credential on a résumé, one more achievement that may tip the scales in their teen's favor. For a lot of parents, it's another example of their child's success in a society that praises accomplishments. Many parents look at the investments of time and money and personal sacrifices they have made over the years and find it difficult to walk away, even if their gut is telling them to. If their child wants out, it can seem like so many resources down the drain. Kids may stay in these sports long after the love for them has dwindled because they recognize how invested their parents are in this endeavor—and quitting won't look good on applications.

One young woman told me that she remained in volleyball far longer than she wanted to, with her mental health suffering significantly because of exhaustion, pressure to excel by her overbearing coaches, and her own maladaptive perfectionism. She would throw up before every game, but she never seriously considered quitting because she didn't want to let her parents down after their years-long financial and personal sacrifices—or, though it was hard to admit, to be viewed as less by them if she was no longer a volleyball star.

It's Not Just Sports

Intense time commitment, financial cost, and pressure to perform well are not limited just to sports. Numerous opportunities exist for extracurricular involvement in a wide range of activities. If your teen is drawn to artistic endeavors, they can engage in music, dance, theater, creative writing, or art, with options in everything from anime to Zumba, all with associated demands of time, effort, emotion, and financial investment. If your child doesn't gravitate toward sports or the arts, they have a myriad of other potential activities to engage in, including robotics, debate teams, science fairs, Math Olympiads, and Model UN. Opportunities exist in student government, interest groups, entrepreneurship, social activism, and volunteering.

For many kids, there is a true sense of passion and joy involved in pursuing activities beyond the school day or a feeling of finding one's people. Often, though, the thought of how a particular activity might look on a college résumé is never far away. Kids (and parents) relate to me that they feel enormous pressure for heavy involvement in extracurriculars. For parents, especially when children are younger, it is driven by social pressure that equates good parenting with the provision of a wide range of enrichment activities and neglect with the opposite—and it continues as their kids grow older.

For teens, taking part in extracurriculars is often motivated by increasing their chances of admission to a highly selective college. Brett, whose story we followed in chapter 7, pursued multiple activities that he thought would look impressive on his application to Duke, including his roles as president of the Chess Club and vice president of the Community Service Club, as well as varsity soccer. Anja, a junior in a high school in northern New Jersey, loves art and has taken multiple classes over the years, spending long hours in the art studio after school. Recently she started entering art competitions and trying to get her paintings shown in local galleries—so that she can stand out and get into a selective art program in college. She's beginning to wonder if it is a good idea, however, as art is no longer the happy place it once was for her. This idea that having a talent for something that you love is not enough, or that doing something for enjoyment only is a waste of time, can trickle down from parents, teachers, and others, bringing the expectation that everything should be taken to the next level, promoted and commodified as part of your shiny admissions package. Hustle culture is an enormous drain on our kids' time, energy, and happiness.

Private Tutoring and Test Prep Courses

Many teens are also squeezing test prep and tutoring into their crammed schedules in an attempt to stand out from the crowd. It is estimated that the number of private test prep and tutoring centers (e.g., Kumon, Sylvan, and Kaplan) more than *tripled* between 1997 and 2022, part of an estimated $24.9 billion U.S. market, and growth in online learning and education support (e.g., Princeton Review, Varsity Tutors, Khan Academy, Tutor.com) has exploded as well.[4] The available services at these centers are broad and include tutoring, test prep, on-demand homework help, enrichment, and skills development (in areas such as coding, engineering, and creative writing). The pressure to engage in these activities starts well before high school, driven by achievement culture that has encroached earlier and earlier in childhood. The perceived needs for tutoring are myriad—helping a child who is struggling with academic material and can't keep up with their daily work in one or more subjects, providing assistance to a child who is striving for straight As, and offering preparation for a multitude of tests to maximize competitiveness, including standardized tests, placement tests for specialized high schools or independent schools, SATs, or ACTs. I know of parents who hired a math tutor for their kindergartener to help him make it into the gifted program or honors track, and high schoolers getting a tutor to improve on an already-exceptional SAT score of 1540.

Ned Johnson is the president and founder of PrepMatters, a Washington, D.C.–based company that offers academic tutoring and standardized test prep. He is also an acclaimed author (and coauthor) of several books on raising self-motivated kids, including *The Self-Driven Child: The Science and Sense of Giving Your Kids More Control over Their Lives* (coauthored with William Stixrud). Ned, a self-described professional "tutor-geek," has worked in the field of academic support since 1993 and has seen profound changes over that time. Ned shared with me that in the past, tutoring and test prep tended to be utilized by two groups: the exceedingly affluent family trying to engineer a path to admission to a highly selective college, and people of varying financial means whose kids were struggling in school.

In recent years, he has noticed a dramatic increase in usage across socioeconomic strata, with many more middle- and upper-middle-class families seeking his company's services, often in support of a child's path to elite schools. And it's not only help with SAT and ACT testing. Often there is a comprehensive plan intended to support students throughout the high school years: standardized test prep, homework assistance, study techniques, coaching, all with an eye to achieving a near-perfect GPA and a smooth college admissions journey in the future. Ned has also seen a steep rise in the number of families enlisting help to *avoid* struggle rather than help with it. He describes it as "prophylactic tutoring," manifest as getting a tutor at the earliest whiff of struggle or putting tutors in place ahead of time to avoid any difficulty on the path to top grades. There has also been a recent surge in the number of families utilizing tutors for unmotivated kids, what Ned describes as "outsourcing the nag." Usually, in these cases, the family's primary objective for the tutor is to ensure that the homework gets completed.

Ned believes that these trends to hire a tutor are largely driven by increasing competition for, and fear about, admissions at highly selective colleges combined with progressive and pervasive grade inflation that makes getting a B in a course feel like a death knell for hopes for admission to the elite college of one's dreams. One family with aspirations for their daughter to go to Princeton flew into a fury with her daughter's teacher and then the school's administration when she, a sophomore, got her first B in a course. They were convinced that her grade would slam the door shut forever to that prestigious school and the future it promised.

It is important to note that while tutoring and test prep assistance can have significant benefits—primarily, helping kids develop their knowledge and skills—they also can have unintended negative consequences. These include a lower sense of student self-efficacy and confidence, increased dependence on assistance to face academic challenges and a parallel decrease in willingness to try to take risks and figure things out, feelings of inadequacy and stigma related to the service provided, an excessive focus on personal performance, and, potentially, an increase in performance anxiety and maladaptive perfectionism. One bright young person I know, who attended summer tutoring sessions prior to their junior year at the strong urging of their well-meaning parents, observed that the tutoring did nothing to raise their SAT scores and was a demoralizing experience overall. They felt as if their great GPA and perfectly solid test scores were deemed not good enough. Parental investment intended to help their child be more successful had the unintended consequence of making them *feel* less successful. So, a word of caution here: You may feel that the tutoring assistance you're supporting is in your child's best interest, aimed at maximizing their options (as the parents of this teen put it); however, you should listen carefully to how they react to the prospect of extra help, as it may not be landing in the way you intended.

The Impact on Teens and Families

Extracurricular activities, particularly when balanced and voluntary, can have a range of potential benefits for kids in areas such as skill development, a sense of competence and self-esteem, social development with friendships and teamwork, and the growth of discipline and perseverance. We've all seen teens brimming with joy and energy as they go about pursuits that they truly love, often with friends and teammates who are equally caught up in the endeavor. Moreover, it's proven that physical activity can be great for mental health. However, an excess of activities, particularly sports that are heavily pressured and competitive, can come with costs like chronic sleep deficits, exhaustion, burnout, and mental health disorders, including depression, anxiety, and eating disorders, as well as overuse injuries and time and financial pressures.[5]

Chronic Sleep Deficit

For many teens, one of the biggest impacts of these overstuffed schedules is inadequate sleep. The recommended amount of sleep is nine to eleven hours per night for six- to thirteen-year-olds, and eight to ten hours for fourteen- to seventeen-year-olds.[6] Yet at every school in which I've conducted research, high schoolers have reported on average getting *six and a half* hours of sleep per school night. And some of them—the especially diligent kids, the ones with AP classes, and those with learning differences—are getting even fewer. Another way to put this in perspective? High school students in my studies, fourteen- to seventeen-year-olds by and large, report getting less sleep each night than first- and second-year medical students—a population that is famous for being overscheduled and sleep deprived.

Too many activities and not enough hours in the day can lead to a lack of sleep, but stress and anxiety can also affect sleep duration and quality. Many teens simply cannot fall asleep—or stay asleep—because their nervous system is constantly activated and they're unable to relax enough to drift into restorative slumber.

From the time my own kids became adolescents, I told them repeatedly that sleep is food for the brain, and this is absolutely true: Deprive it of this nourishment, and negative consequences will follow. A child who is getting six and a half hours of sleep a night is cognitively and emotionally compromised, experiencing decreases in memory, attention, executive function, abstract thinking, behavioral control, and mood. One famous study showed that the effect on hand-eye coordination of staying up for twenty-four hours was comparable to having a blood alcohol level of 0.10 percent.[7] In the U.S., this would be viewed as too impaired to drive. Another study examined the impact of restricted sleep in adolescents for five nights (6.5 hours per night, the same amount that the students surveyed averaged) on cognition and found a marked decrease in attention, alertness, and quiz performance.[8] Chronic inadequate sleep has also been linked to a number of health risks, including obesity, metabolic dysfunction, hypertension, anxiety, depression, and risk-taking behaviors.[9]

A Threat to Mental Health

In a 2013 paper titled "I Can, Therefore I Must," researcher Suniya Luthar examined the association between the number of hours spent in extracurricular activities and depression/anxiety in eighth graders and high school juniors and seniors. To her surprise, she found no direct correlation; more hours didn't automatically translate to higher levels of depression/anxiety. What she did find, however, was that the *nature* of the activities correlated with mental health conditions. If they were highly competitive and kids felt pressure, criticism, and overly high expectations from adults, their mental health suffered.[10] Luthar noted that this pressure to succeed in extracurricular activities can come from parents *and* also from outside the family in the form of coaches and teachers who are invested in having their athletes or students excel.

Another source of pressure observed by Luthar was peer group comparisons. Teens often look to see how their competitors are faring, measuring their performances against their own—especially easy to do, or hard to avoid, with social media. Teens frequently want to see who made the team or who won the star role in the school musical, and they rank themselves accordingly. Luthar advocated for a balance between structured and unstructured time, noting that moderate involvement in *meaningful* activities was protective for mental health.

A number of sports and activities that teens are often involved in are associated with elevated risk for eating disorders, especially as athletes become more immersed in competitions. These include those where body appearance is important, such as gymnastics, figure skating, and ballet, as well as speed or endurance sports including swimming, track, and cross-country. Pressure to lose weight and body-shaming have been all-too-common features of coaching in these sports.

Rising Burnout in Teens and Parents

Burnout has been the focus of intense study and attention, primarily in healthcare and other high-stress work settings, and is therefore less commonly associated with kids.[11] The term was coined by American psychologist Herbert Freudenberger in the 1970s, based on his work observing staff stress in free health clinics. In its *International Classification of Diseases, 11th Revision,* the World Health Organization defines burnout as "a syndrome conceptualized as resulting from chronic workplace stress that has not been successfully managed." However, burnout can just as easily be caused by the stresses and demands of school and a taxing schedule of extracurriculars, leading to a constant state of emotional and physical exhaustion. In the face of such pressures, there is insufficient time to slow down, relax, and connect with other people, and burnout is an almost inevitable outcome for kids, certainly, but also relatedly for parents too. The pressure of kids' overscheduled lives is a family affair.

Social psychologist Christina Maslach, a pioneer in the study of burnout who continues her work today, has characterized burnout as having three dimensions: emotional exhaustion, depersonalization, and a diminished sense of personal accomplishment.[12]

- Emotional exhaustion can manifest through chronic fatigue, irritability, and a constant state of feeling overwhelmed. It's the kind of fatigue that doesn't go away, even if you manage to get a good night's sleep, and can leave you drained and wondering how you can possibly make it through the mountain of things you have to do. For teens, it can be a feeling of exhaustion and stress that just won't let up.

- Depersonalization is characterized by callousness and decreased empathy. You and your teen might experience emotional numbness or disconnection, or feel that you're just going through the motions of your life without really living it.

- A diminished sense of personal accomplishment can appear as negative self-talk, doubting one's competence, and a loss of pride in achievements large and small—which can make it difficult to muster the energy to get anything done.

It is important to recognize, though, that these are not the only manifestations or characteristics of burnout, which also include negativity, pessimism, cynicism, and short-temperedness. Together, the symptoms of burnout can make a packed schedule and excessive demands feel all the more overwhelming—which can lead to a toxic cycle that increases and prolongs burnout.

In 2024, then-surgeon general Vivek Murthy shone a light on the stresses that parents face in an advisory titled *Parents Under Pressure: The U.S. Surgeon General's Advisory on the Mental Health and Well-Being of Parents.*[13] The report found that "41 percent of parents say that they are so stressed that they cannot function and 48 percent say that most days their stress is completely overwhelming." Several factors play a part in this, including an increase in demands on their time due to work and family responsibilities, which "can contribute to work-family conflict, burnout, and stress." The report also highlights that "a modern practice of time-intensive parenting and contemporary expectations around childhood achievement may contribute further to the stressors faced by parents."[14] In some cases, living with such high levels of stress can translate into mental illness, such as anxiety and depression, for parents, which can then affect children, contributing to higher rates of poor general and mental health and behavioral and developmental problems.[15]

When we are drained by the demands of life, whether we are parents being pulled in multiple directions or kids with overpacked schedules, we find it harder to cope on a daily basis because burnout affects our "window of tolerance." This concept, created by psychiatrist Daniel J. Siegel and explored in his 1999 book, *The Developing Mind,* describes the zone in which each of us can function at our best, even when confronted by life's stressors. Within this "window," our nervous system is regulated, and we feel calm, present, and grounded. However, chronic stress and burnout can narrow our window of tolerance, leaving us less able to handle life's everyday demands. When this happens, a single negative event or an accumulation of incidents can be overwhelming, activating the nervous system and bringing on a cascade of intense emotions that we feel powerless to stop. For example, being benched in the middle of a basketball game or being stuck in traffic after a disappointing floor routine at an out-of-town gymnastics competition can cause a flood of anger, frustration, sadness, or shame.

Parents have spoken to me with concern about their teens having meltdowns or temper tantrums, when they just seem to lose their ability to regulate their emotions. Some parents have added that they too have felt this way on many occasions. Other people, often family members, can become unwitting targets of uncontrolled anger or frustration when burnout has caused a diminished window of tolerance. Later in the chapter, I'll offer some practical tools for parents and teens alike for navigating and managing burnout.

Compromised Relationships

Strong parental and peer connections have been consistently shown to be associated with better mental health in teens.[16] Unfortunately, overscheduling can be a major threat to those relationships, particularly when high-pressure, competitive, and time-intensive activities dominate. For many families, together time consists of parents shuttling a child from activity to activity, which hardly counts as high-quality interaction. The burnout that can accrue from this frantic collective activity can manifest in frazzled nerves and short tempers in both parents and children, further compromising closeness. Sometimes parents find themselves taking on the role of coach for their teens involved in sports, becoming overly invested in or critical about their child's performance. This can lead to conflict and blurred boundaries in the parent-child relationship and can increase stress for the child. When schedules are busy, family dinners, where deeper, more relaxed connection can occur, can become infrequent or in some situations can completely disappear. Many parents have shared stories of dinner grabbed with their teens in the car on the way to or from rehearsals or practice. The idea of every family member being at home, or even in the same place, at dinner time is laughable for them—though something that they yearn for.

Parents caught in the trap of their kids' frenzied activities may lose opportunities to invest time in their own pursuits, interests, and relationships, potentially building resentment about what they are giving up and increasing pressure on their kids to excel. Time with friends may also be heavily curtailed, and friend groups can become narrowed to fellow parents of teammates or participants in that specific activity. Isaac, a dad I know, with two teens involved in competitive soccer, shared with me that he and his partner haven't had a "real date," as he puts it, in years. "Sure, we grab food together once in a while, but the thought of us spending a relaxed evening out, maybe dinner and a movie, some extended, focused time together—well, it's just not happening. We've accepted that it's the season we're in. But I don't love it. And I don't think it's good for us. But what can you do?" A colleague told me that when her teen quit tennis, she and her husband realized they didn't have any friends left who weren't part of the competitive tennis circuit. Their whole world had been caught up in their daughter's sport.

Lack of Time for Free Play

All of this hectic extracurricular and structured activity has led to a lack of time for kids to engage in free play starting at earlier and earlier ages. In a society that values productivity, this may not be perceived by many as a great loss. However, free play is crucial to human experience—it is an important activity in which kids can enjoy simple fun, no pressure attached, and it plays a fundamental role in their social development on the path to adulthood. As researcher Peter Gray has said, "One of the major functions of play is it's how children learn how to take charge of their own activities, to initiate and decide what to do, to negotiate with their playmates about what they're going to do. To create the rules or modify the rules as they go along to make the play fun and interesting. . . . When adults take over the activity, as happens in adult organized sports, then you're completely destroying that major function of play, which is for children to learn how to do things themselves and solve their own problems."[17]

In chapter 10, I'll explore further the role of unstructured play as it relates to autonomy, meaning, and belonging—all elements that can help your child thrive in the face of overwhelming academic and extracurricular schedules.

What Can a Parent Do?

It may seem that there is little you can do in the face of societal pressure when it comes to your child's extracurriculars. But acknowledging the problem of overscheduling coupled with relentless competition around the clock is an important first step. Deciding to turn your attention to addressing it as best you can is already a positive move forward. Parents have substantial opportunities to change their children's—and their own—lives for the better; here are some strategies that I hope are useful.

Schedule family time first and stress the importance of family/friends. It has been estimated that by the time your child turns eighteen, you will have spent 90 percent of the total time you'll have with them in your lifetime. What a striking point to consider—and all the more reason to be thoughtful about creating opportunities to connect with your child. Rather than assuming, or hoping, that family time and time with friends will simply occur, schedule it like you would any other activity—and aim to get it on the calendar first so that you can plan around it rather than squeezing it into an already chock-a-block week. Do your best to instill boundaries so that family time stays in place. Model to your kids ways that you prioritize time with them. If you have, for example, standing family dinners on Sundays, say no to other potential commitments. Consider instituting a no-screens policy for times you spend together so that you can truly be present with one another. Try to emphasize downtime as well, spending time with your kids in low-key activities like walking the dog, throwing a frisbee in the backyard, or going for ice cream. Remember that you're blocking out time on your calendar rather than adding additional activities.

Prioritize sleep. Ensuring that everyone in your family gets enough sleep can make a big difference in your lives. Think about what time each person needs to wake up in the morning and then count backwards to set a bedtime that provides the requisite hours of sleep. While it may seem unlikely or impossible that your teen will be asleep by 10:00 p.m. or even 11:00 p.m. during the school week, setting a firm, but reasonable goal will help everyone (including you) get more sleep into their lives. There may be pushback in the beginning, but hold the line. There were times when my daughters wanted to stay up late studying, usually the night before an exam. My most persuasive argument against this idea was that anything they learned in that late-night hour or two wouldn't be worth it—their lack of sleep would compromise their cognitive functioning and their exam performance overall. I also told them that if they wanted to get up early to study they could, but they never made that choice!

Have a "no screens in bedrooms" policy after a certain hour and make sure your kids abide by it. It likely won't be easy, but after all, you're probably the person who is footing the bill for their technology, so you get the final say. Encourage your child to have a wind-down routine away from screens before they go to sleep, one that their body will begin to associate with relaxation. It could be deep breathing, listening to music, or reading an old-fashioned paper-and-ink book. The bottom line is: Get serious about sleep.

Help your child make reasonable choices about extracurriculars. While respecting your teen's (and child's and preteen's) autonomy, provide guidance if you think they are overextending themselves. Given the culture that they've grown up in, many teens think it's completely normal to be scheduled every minute of the day, so you may have to let them know that it's okay to pull back. Explore with them why they are choosing an activity. Is it because they have a genuine interest in it or do they think it will look good on their future college application? In his application to Duke, Brett probably didn't improve his chances by having more than a dozen activities listed. Be aware, too, of your own reasons for signing your kids up for one activity versus another. I've heard stories of parents enlisting their eight-year-olds in fencing lessons—so that their child's college application will stand out from others' a decade down the line.

Do research on club sports/travel teams. Be aware of what you, as a parent, are signing up for before encouraging, or allowing, your child to get involved in club sports. This isn't a decision to be taken lightly, given what it might entail. Ask some questions before you say yes to your eager child or teen. What is the time commitment each week? Is attendance at all practices and games mandatory? Is the commitment for just one season or does it extend over the year? What are the expectations for parents? How about the financial commitment? Does the sport have heavy costs for equipment? What are the anticipated costs for any travel?

Nowadays, many teams have contracts for parents and older kids to sign, so be sure to read a contract in full—and have your child read it too so they fully understand their obligations. Once you're aware of what your family's participation would look like, you can decide whether it's the right choice for you. Do you have the financial/energy/time resources to commit? Think about and discuss together what you want your family life to look like—taking into account siblings who will likely be affected even if they're not playing the sport. Are you willing to sacrifice regular family dinners and get-togethers with friends? If you do decide to go ahead, make a pact to take it season by season or year by year and reassess as a family. Agree ahead of time that if it's not working for everyone you'll step back.

Recently, Kristin, the Minnesota ice hockey player, decided that she had had enough of intense competition after her high school team completed its season. It was imposing too much of a burden on her. She didn't want to continue with her club team but was hesitant to talk to her parents, fearing they would be disappointed in her. It turned out that they were happy to reassess and felt relieved by her decision, knowing the physical and mental toll it had taken on her. They reassured her that they wanted her to be happy and that her health and well-being were the most important thing.

Make hard choices. Sometimes you'll have to take a stand and prioritize what's important in your family life while balancing the commitments your teen has made to an after-school activity. Attending Grandma's eightieth birthday party and missing a practice or a game may get your child benched—but honoring and celebrating Grandma as a family is more important. What messages are you sending if you sacrifice important life events for a sport?

Don't be afraid to say no if you sense it's not what you're looking for as a family. One parent I know was asked by her ten-year-old daughter if she could join a travel soccer team with her friend. When the mom asked, "Do you know what travel soccer is?" the girl responded, "It's like the Yankees, but for soccer." "Yes," said the mom, "except the Yankees players don't drag their entire family with them to every game." They decided not to do travel soccer, and the girl happily joined a local soccer league instead.

Likewise, Kurt and Jennifer, the parents I introduced you to in chapter 8, have chosen a different path for after-school activities and sports for their son Peter and themselves. While he is a good athlete, they enrolled him in low-key, low-cost rec leagues in his community with friends from his neighborhood. Practice takes place before their game each week. There are no thirty-minute drives to distant suburbs for practices, no weekend trips to other cities for tournaments. No heavy pressure to win or intense criticism from coaches, just a good game with teammates. With this, family dinners at home are the norm more nights than not, and Peter loves having the freedom to ride his bike to his friends' houses after school instead of being ferried to and from practice. They are free to play together and unwind from their school day without the constant supervision of adults—something that fewer and fewer kids are experiencing in their overscheduled lives.

If your child is involved in sports or other competitive activities, be their biggest supporter. As mentioned earlier, Suniya Luthar found that excessive pressure and criticism from parents (and other adults) relating to extracurricular activities was associated with depression and anxiety in teens. Bear this in mind if your child is involved in a sports team (or other activities), and try to support them win or lose. Leave the coaching and critiques to the coaches or teachers. Just as with academics, you should strive to provide a low-pressure supportive zone at home with regard to extracurriculars. If the coaches seem too intense or overly critical, then provide them feedback or consider pulling your child out if it becomes too extreme and feels as if it goes against your values. The mother of baseball player Jordan wished that she had asked the coach to scale back the intensity before her son needed Tommy John surgery, but by then it was too late.

A parent told me about witnessing a softball game where a coach on the opposing team stood over the eight-year-old kids and screamed at them, berating them for their performance. No one stepped in to intervene. That kind of coaching behavior should be seen as unacceptable rather than common—and parents should feel that they can call it out.

Encourage rest and recovery time at home. Some families, including those who aren't religious, have instituted a day of rest, a sabbath of sorts in which work of any kind is not done, and some have made it a screen-free day as well, promoting rest, relaxation, recovery, and connection.[18] See if it makes sense for your family, starting out with a shorter time period at first if necessary.

Take action on behalf of your child. Sometimes, even if you've been intentional about your family's involvement in extracurriculars, you'll likely need to intervene if things become too intense. Boosters, or parent volunteers, of a high school theater program banded together with good results after rehearsals went on too late for too long. The school was putting on a showstopping version of *Hairspray*, and in the last couple of weeks before opening night, rehearsals had gone until 10:00 p.m. It was exhausting for the kids, who had been at school all day, as well as for their parents, who had to collect them afterward. After the show closed, the boosters initiated an aptly named "postmortem" with the director, during which they said, "What can we do to avoid late rehearsals ever, ever again?" They were gentle about it, but they also revealed to her the enormous toll that the crushing schedule had had upon the kids—how many of them had gotten sick and missed school after the intensity of the show. The boosters had come with data in hand about how crucial sleep is for the developing adolescent brain. The drama director agreed to a hard stop at 9:00 p.m. for all future rehearsals. This was a case where a do-or-die mentality had taken hold, and where the cost of the sacrifice and the absolute need to bring balance into the lives of kids and families were crystal clear. Not every situation is quite this clear, but this question needs to be kept in mind: When does an enrichment opportunity veer into the territory of harm? It can be subtle—a bit too much of a good thing—or dramatic, as in the above example, where kids are being sickened through a ridiculous amount of demands and are suffering the consequences. Be ready to step in—and join with other parents—as necessary.

Strategies for Managing Burnout

Burnout is incredibly common in parents, and while it is critically important to take steps to reduce the sources of burnout in your life, it can also be helpful to know how to manage it when it occurs so you can be your best self in the face of life's inevitable stresses. In addition to the powerful cognitive restructuring techniques that I teach to students and physicians (and shared with you in chapter 6), I teach simple skills designed to help manage the impact of stress and maintain or regain calm and composure and some level of positivity and optimism when things are tough.

Some two decades ago, I found myself constantly stressed by pressures in my professional life that kept me at a high simmer and pushed me outside my window of tolerance. For seven years, I had consistently put in a seventy-five-hour workweek as a pediatric clinician and faculty member at UCLA, becoming used to the unrelenting schedule and multitude of responsibilities that came with it. It was only when my family and I moved to St. Louis, and I to a different job, that I realized how burned out I had been. At the time, I was somewhat aware that my stress and fatigue sometimes leaked out and affected my family—and that work was getting my better self. I wasn't an ogre at home, but I didn't quite rise to the standards that I had set for myself at work, where I was more patient, positive, and understanding. By the time I pulled into my driveway at the end of a long day in which stressors had mounted and accumulated, my window of tolerance was often a tiny porthole. Perhaps you can relate to this. Some of you—and your kids—may be in a similar situation, brought on by the incessant demands of a hectic and exhausting schedule.

I realized that I needed to come up with a tool to help myself regulate my emotions better in the face of escalating stress and to manage my overactivated nervous system. First, I decided to find a common and predictable stressor in my life where I could develop and hone this skill. It hit me immediately—grocery lines would be the perfect practice ground, as they drove me completely crazy. Invariably, I would choose the slow line, then leap to a faster-moving line, which would then become the slow line, my stress levels building all the while. Rushed and frantic and fuming inside, I would scout the various lines to try to reverse my luck—which rarely happened. When I finally made it to the cashier, my stress would be at an all-time high. Perhaps you recognize this scenario, or something akin to it, such as sitting in traffic or waiting for videos that take forever to load. We all have stressors that push us to the edge of our capacity to deal with the situation at hand with a semblance of self-control.

In order to increase your teen's capacity—and your own—to manage stress and effectively regulate emotions even when burned out, I propose a solution: grocery-line mindfulness. It's simple and effective, and it's based on an acceptance that we all have days when we are stretched to the limit and require a skill that keeps us functioning smoothly, despite everything. Here's how it works:

- Notice that you are entering a potentially difficult situation and monitor yourself for signs of stress: the tightening of your jaw, a feeling of dread or looming disaster, or butterflies in your stomach. This is your body's stress response and it's natural—but keep an eye on it.
- Create the tiniest space in your mind, or awareness, and then, in that space, make your reaction to the situation or the feeling

a choice. Remind yourself that you do not have to spiral into frustration or anger or panic, for you know that it won't help the situation at all.

- Breathe deeply and accept that you can't control everything and that you are exactly where you need to be, even if it is the absolute longest and slowest grocery line of all time.

The beautiful thing about this technique is that as you practice it, its effectiveness deepens and expands. You can carry it with you wherever you go. Maybe it's 9:00 p.m. and you've just made it home after work meetings, having picked up one child from dance practice along the way, then hurried to catch the last thirty minutes of your other child's hockey game. All you want to do is take a warm bath and have an early night, but there's dinner to heat up and homework to be done. As you feel your heart racing and tension rising, you know you're about to explode—but with the grocery line mindfulness tool you can create a tiny space in your mind and choose your reaction. You can breathe deeply in and out to keep yourself calm and not succumb to irritability born of exhaustion and frustration. Think of the difference that this choice can make.

In addition, here are some other simple techniques that you and your teen can use to help with feelings of burnout and stress:

- **Cultivate positive emotions.** A simple approach to feel more positive emotions is a practice called Three Good Things. Keep a journal handy, perhaps on a night table next to your bed, and at bedtime write down three good things that happened that day. It could be a big thing—like a great team effort and a big basketball win—or something small, like "the burrito I had at lunch was just spectacular!" It's a practice that reinforces the notion—and truth—that good things, big and small, happen a lot, even in the midst of challenging times—and if you find yourself doubting it at any time, you'll have the data ready to back it up.

- **Promote optimism.** As I wrote in chapter 7, it used to be thought that optimism and pessimism were fixed traits, but this has turned out to be untrue. You can work to become more of a glass-half-full person, and you can engage in activities that can promote optimism in your family. One practice I like is called appreciative inquiry, which counters a common tendency we humans have to tell stories of challenge, difficulty, and frustration when we are stressed. At times, it feels good to vent in this way; however, if these are the main or only stories that you're telling, or that are being told around you, ask yourself what kind of environment or worldview they are creating. Be sure to tell, and ask for, stories of grace, beauty, self-efficacy, courage, or humor. These stories are all around you, but they can become lost in the midst of life's stresses and pressure. Try to model this for your teen.
- **Practice gratitude.** Regularly practicing and expressing gratitude has been shown to improve well-being. Common practices include journaling, having a gratitude board, or engaging in family gratitude rituals (such as "Share one thing you are grateful for today").

As we reach the end of the chapter, I'd like to share with you a simple success story. You may remember Daniela and her friends from the beginning of the chapter who were trying to enjoy a summer potluck—but their kids' activities got in the way. Recently, Daniela told me that her friend group had done some deep reflection on what they wanted for their families going forward. It looked different for all of them, but she and four other families decided to speak with their kids' soccer coach and ask for fewer tournaments next year and one less practice a week. To their surprise, their coach said yes. It felt like a sweet victory—and they already have the potluck on the calendar.

Chapter 10

Giving Kids More Control, More Choice, and Opportunities to Find Connection, Meaning, and Joy

Wren was a sophomore student in a suburban high school in the Midwest, where they were miserable and profoundly depressed. Each day they sat through their classes, feeling little connection to the material as their teachers lectured and handed out endless worksheets. They had limited elective opportunities or time to explore their own interests. At the end of the day, they came home exhausted, but there was still work to be done. The homework load was overwhelming, and Wren felt as if they were "being buried under a huge pile of rubble." Over the course of the semester, they fell further and further behind, accruing what they described as an ever-growing "homework debt," until they felt as if they were in "a Titanic-sized boat filling with water with only one shoe to use to bail it out." The overall effect, as Wren described it, was one of meaningless, joyless drudgery, that left them feeling dull and numb.

Wren's mother, Claudia, an educator herself, did what she could to help them manage the onslaught of material. Wren had been diagnosed with ADHD in middle school, and Claudia helped them with executive function tasks like navigating the school's online platform, creating systems for tracking schoolwork and assignments, and helping them with worksheets, doing her best to just keep them afloat. When signs of depression emerged, Claudia moved quickly to get Wren mental health care. Wren appreciated all of her help and care, describing home as "sweet relief" at the end of the day, but said that "demons" from school followed them there and lingered. This academic exertion consumed the lion's share of their family time, and despite all of her efforts, Claudia felt helpless and powerless to protect her child from the educational system.

Wren would perform fairly well on exams, but late or missing worksheets were figured in as a significant portion of the grade, so their GPA fell below 3.0. They didn't feel like their grades were a measure of their worth and value (embracing their mom's message to them, "You are not your grades"), but they worried that any future aspirations for a successful life were being compromised. Would any decent college accept them? It was hard to be hopeful about the future.

Everything changed in the summer between sophomore and junior year when Wren worked as a volunteer intern in a camp program at the local zoo. Their mood brightened immediately. They were doing what *they* wanted to do in a setting that they had chosen. They worked alongside "amazing" people who shared common interests in animals and education. Overall, they performed relatively menial tasks, sweeping floors, taking little kids for bathroom breaks, and making sure the campers had their art projects to take home when parents picked them up. But at the end of the day they felt like they had accomplished something worthwhile and that they were part of something bigger than themselves. The experience was transformational; Wren blossomed, and Claudia was thrilled and relieved.

But the positive effects didn't last. Soon after the start of their junior year, the grind of school took its toll, and their depression reemerged. Wren and their mom ground through the academic year, buoyed intermittently by evening education programs sponsored by the zoo, but overall, Wren's mental health suffered. It wasn't until the following summer that their depression symptoms receded when they returned to the zoo to carry out a paid internship. As part of their work, they designed a program to promote the planting of native seeds in local yards, participated in the care of beetles, and ultimately went on a field trip to release them into the wild. Despite sometimes starting work at 7:00 a.m. and not getting home until 10:00 p.m., they felt energized, alive, and joyous. They had discovered something that they cared about, that they were good at, and that gave a shape and purpose to their days. Finding meaning was critical to their dramatic improvement in mental health.

The Importance of Meaning and Joy

One of the key components of the interventions that I led at SLU to improve our medical students' mental health was to create opportunities for them to find meaning and joy in their lives. I had thought it would be important for them to orient their lives to something bigger than passing courses and getting through medical school. We were able to accomplish this by freeing up time for electives and encouraging students to get involved in activities that they cared deeply about—for the sake of the activities themselves. I imagine it was the first time they had received such directions in years. Students jumped in wholeheartedly, and the range of activities that they chose was as striking and unique as the students themselves. One shadowed a doula. She was so moved by the experience that she created an elective for students to be trained as doulas, following women through their pregnancy and deliveries, providing support and finding, in the process, fulfillment and meaning of their own. Another group of students wanted to start a student-run, faculty-supervised clinic for unhoused people, but upper administration nixed the idea because of concerns about ensuring faculty staffing. Rather than give up their quest, students considered what services they could provide without faculty supervision. They landed on cleaning and taking care of people's feet, as foot issues can be a devastating problem for the unhoused. Students would sit and provide care, engaging in conversation, learning about people's lives and struggles, giving comfort where they could—and feeling good about themselves in the process. It was clear that our students' mental health rallied after our interventions, and I felt sure that their embrace of meaningful activities that they had chosen themselves and that brought them joy had played a huge role.

The Role of Self-Determination Theory

Some years later, I learned about a theory that seemed to back this up—self-determination theory. I believe that it explains, to a great degree, the efficacy of our initiative at SLU, as well as the improvement in mental health and well-being for Wren, and that it can also help inform how we address the current mental health crisis in teens.

Self-determination theory (SDT) was created by Edward Deci and Richard Ryan and has been the subject of more than a thousand research studies.[1] The theory posits that people are most motivated and function at their best when three basic psychological needs are met: autonomy, competence, and relatedness.

- Autonomy as defined by Deci and Ryan is not freedom to do whatever you want. Rather, it involves being able, or empowered, to make choices that are voluntary rather than forced or coerced and that are consistent with your personal values.
- Competence is having the feeling that you are effective and capable in some sphere in your life.
- Relatedness is having strong relationships and feeling deeply connected to others, having a sense of belonging.

When one's needs for autonomy, competence, and relatedness are satisfied, intrinsic motivation (our inner drive) increases; when these needs are thwarted, motivation tends to be extrinsic in nature (driven, for example, by grades or awards) and declines. Intrinsic motivation has many benefits that should make it attractive to parents and educators—improved learning outcomes, deeper engagement, improved creativity, enhanced problem-solving, greater persistence and resilience, and healthier relationships. What's more, meeting the three basic psychological needs of autonomy, competence, and relatedness has also been shown in multiple studies to increase well-being and decrease depression and anxiety.[2]

With the introduction of less classwork, more electives, and the opportunity to collaborate with one another, the students at SLU thrived, experiencing advances in each area. They could decide what activities to take up outside of the core curriculum, and we encouraged them to engage in pursuits that they cared about and found meaning in rather than just padding their résumés. They had the opportunity to build competence in areas of personal interest, often gaining knowledge in new subject areas and fresh insights into their own strengths. At a class meeting where we talked about the ongoing curricular changes, one student who had struggled with the intense academic demands of the first two years of med school said, with tears in her eyes, "Dr. Slavin, you gave me a way to feel good about myself." Student relatedness also improved as the move to a pass/fail grading system allowed students to view one another as collaborators in their academic endeavors, as being all in this together, rather than competitors. They worked side by side, often along with faculty, deepening personal connections and creating community where it had been previously lacking.

Looking back, I believe these elements not only were responsible for the dramatic drop in depression and anxiety rates but also contributed to something more: student flourishing. Depression and anxiety rates decreased significantly in our students, but what was especially striking was that the number of students with *very* low depression and anxiety scores skyrocketed. The graph below provides a before-and-after snapshot.[*3]

The light gray bars represent student depression before the curriculum changes, and the dark gray bars represent depression rates after the changes. Looking at the dark gray bars, you can see the decrease in

---

* Originally published in Slavin, Stuart J., and John T. Chibnall. "Finding the why, changing the how: improving the mental health of medical students, residents, and physicians." *Academic Medicine* 91, no. 9 (2016): 1194–1196. Reproduced with permission.

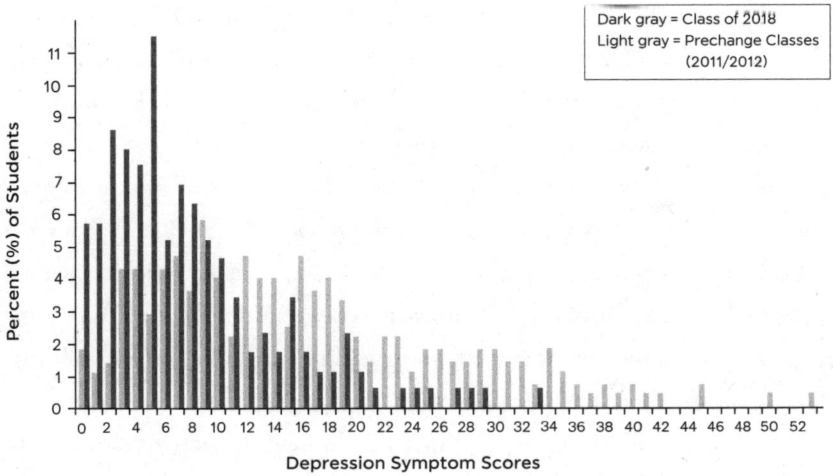

students with high scores on the depression axis as well as the huge increase on the left of students with low to very low scores when compared to the light gray bars.

And it wasn't just the numbers that bore this out; you could feel the newfound energy and joy in the hallways and the classrooms as students went about their days engaged with the faculty and one another in classes and learning communities, in their electives, and in volunteer activities. We heard more laughter and saw more smiles, and there just seemed to be less tension in the air. In the years since I left SLU, I have encountered former students who shared that they learned something in these self-driven pursuits that made them, in the long run, better doctors. They were able to see the bigger picture. What may have started with examining the feet of an unhoused person developed over time into a doctoring approach that takes the whole patient and their unique circumstances into account.

Self-Determination Theory and Teens' Lives Today

When kids' lives are examined through the lens of self-determination theory, meaning, and joy, one can see why so many kids, and their families, are suffering. The persistent pursuit of grades and scores to gain admission to a highly selective college is for many a meaningless, grueling quest, one that consumes a vast amount of their time and energy, both at school and at home. There is a world of difference between an intrinsic motivation fueled by a genuine desire to learn, explore, and grow as a human and an extrinsic motivation to achieve narrow goals that are not necessarily your own. It's safe to say that nearly all of us have noted firsthand this contrast in our own life experiences.

There is strong evidence that intrinsic motivation among teens has been declining for decades[4] and may well be contributing to a deterioration in their mental health. Self-determination theory states that autonomy, competence, and relatedness are fundamental universal human needs, applicable to every age across the lifespan, including childhood and adolescence, and yet many kids, both at school and in extracurricular activities, have few opportunities to experience any of them or find meaning in what they do. It's not surprising that their mental health, well-being, and happiness are on the decline.

Childhood, and especially the teen years, is a time in which kids should be figuring out a sense of self, what they have a passion for, where they feel connection, and what their beliefs and values are in a process called identity formation, yet the relentless chase of scores, grades, and achievement undermines this critically important developmental task. In the end, they may find themselves at the academic finish line not really knowing who they are or what they want out of life. The path to flourishing as an adult begins with figuring yourself out, using your internal compass to find direction, and navigating with joy and passion. As a parent, it is essential to keep self-determination theory and meaning-making in mind as you help your kid discover their developing self. In the next section, I'll discuss what this guidance might look like in the life of your teen.

Autonomy

Most teens have very limited autonomy at school—a little, perhaps, in choosing their classes, especially in the higher grades in private schools, and little to none in choosing their teachers or what or when they learn, and how—other than the freedom to choose not to learn much at all—which some kids, particularly boys, opt for. While they may have some control over their choices of after-school activities, they generally have little say in how those activities are conducted and led. Often their choices are driven not by a passion to do or learn something but rather by a perceived necessity to build their résumé for their college application. I've heard stories of teens helping out at local soup kitchens or aiding seniors with technology advice, not through a sense of empathy or community, but just to check a box—and when they've accomplished that goal, they leave and move on to the next one with no thought of staying to lend a hand because they are needed or making a difference.

Often their choices are directed by adults. I know of a sixteen-year-old girl who was eager to walk dogs after school but who was persuaded by a teacher to take coding classes instead. "They'll round out your applications," she was told. Kids may feel little or no sense of autonomy if their parents are overinvolved in decisions about extracurricular activities and all the logistics that they entail, which can spill over into how their unscheduled time—if any—is spent. Beth, a junior high student, was pressured by her Ivy League alum parents to participate in lacrosse, a niche sport that they felt could boost her college applications. Reluctantly, she acquiesced, hating the experience but remaining in the sport to pacify her mom and dad.

Many teens find themselves on such a controlled path toward college success that they aren't allowed or expected to try anything else. I've heard parents say, "Your only job right now is to focus on school"—which is all very well, but it leaves a great swath of their child's inner and outer world unexplored, which not only is limiting but can feel claustrophobic. It also sends the message that the teen needs only to focus on themselves, their own journey, their own success, which can result in self-centered and entitled kids. It turns out that greater autonomy can create space for kids to be more selfless and generous on their path to identity formation.

Given the overly restricted nature of many teens' lives, it's no wonder that so many of them are compulsively drawn to the digital world, where they can experience what feels like almost complete autonomy—though in reality it is dictated and managed by complex and insidious algorithms designed to captivate attention. Still, it represents a space of freedom from overreaching parents, coaches, and teachers. It can feel like a world of one's own.

Competence

Today's teens, despite the outward success that many of them seem to display, are rarely able to experience a sense of competence. They are constantly getting the message that they need to do more and do it better—whether it's AP classes, extracurriculars, internships, or college applications. And with social media, the comparison isn't just to kids on your block or in your school, for videos and memes capture and display outsize accomplishments of kids across the country boasting about GPAs, SAT scores, and awesome college acceptances. It is easy to feel as if you don't measure up, no matter how well you do, as someone else is always doing better. An overemphasis on obtaining perfect scores has escalated in ways that may baffle older generations, who recall the days when a 4.0 GPA was the highest you could get. They may wonder what a GPA of 4.73 even means. And why are rising GPAs failing to produce more feelings of competence? It is due, I would argue, to the simultaneous rises in maladaptive perfectionism, toxic comparison, and performance as identity that I described in chapters 5 and 6, fostered by a culture of relentless and competitive measuring, sorting, and ranking. For many teens, it feels as if the goal posts are constantly moving—there are always more ways to strive to be perfect. Not only must they be straight-A students in every subject, but they're hearing loud and clear the message, from both the achievement culture and college admissions committees, that they also have to be a state champion athlete, national youth poet laureate, or award-winning scientist. And when they're not, they feel less than—or incompetent.

Fifteen-year-old Marly explained it like this: "You study every night until 1:00 a.m. for weeks and get an A minus on a history exam, a class you don't even like, and you feel like you failed. Even though your mom says, 'Great job!' you can see that disappointment in her face that she's trying to hide. And then you're figuring out what you've got to do now to pull your GPA back up because you need to be perfect, so you're doing extra credit even though you don't have time and you've got a swim meet coming up and you want to practice more, otherwise you won't make states. It never stops. And no matter what you do, you never feel like you're good enough."

Relatedness

Too often, education (and the school day overall) lacks opportunities for meaningful connection with others. Some teachers may engage in interactive teaching, but there's a tendency for the same kids to volunteer answers and/or get called upon. The rest are likely to remain passive and disengaged for hour upon hour of class time. While I've observed wonderfully innovative approaches in teaching, the existing system tends not to support them, in part, as I've discussed, because of stringent state requirements that put pressure on teachers to "teach to the test," which limits opportunities for more collaborative, experiential learning. Meaningful connection between students can occur, but it's often tinged with competition as they compete for grades or places in selective colleges. It's hard to experience trust or be vulnerable with others in such a dog-eat-dog world. Overscheduling and the continuous shuttling to various after-school activities can limit opportunities for connection too. Often teens are too busy for meals or real conversations with parents and family members, leading to feelings of disconnection and even loneliness. Very often teens maintain friendships via text or social media platforms, which lack the depth of real-life relationships and can lead to teens missing the opportunity to develop the social skills that they'll need in their adult lives, both socially and professionally.

Let's return to a couple of stories from earlier in the book and examine them through the lens of autonomy, competence, and relatedness. In chapter 2, you met Jason, our high school student from the Bay Area whose existence was a relentless series of classes, test prep courses, and extracurricular activities like Model UN prescribed by his parents. His life was severely lacking in all three pillars of self-determination theory.

He had virtually no autonomy, and while he achieved some academic success, it didn't fill him with a sense of competence in the same way it would have if the achievement was related to something that he really cared about. Relatedness also suffered in his life as all the frenzied activity designed to maximize his GPA, standardized test scores, and ultimately college acceptance left him with no real time for developing and maintaining close friendships, and as his depression grew he shied away from social contact.

Contrast Jason's story with that of the students in the AP Language and Composition class of Andrea Vescelius, our innovative teacher from chapter 8, whose embrace of self-determination theory profoundly influenced and enhanced their experience. They had an unprecedented level of autonomy in what and how they learned, which was tied to their personal interests. As they progressed in the class, they felt a growing sense of competence in something they cared about, whether it was a new language, the stock market, or the cosmos. Rather than focusing on and chasing a final grade in the course, they were able to celebrate their own personal growth and mastery. In addition, with the small group learning that occurred regularly, they developed a real rapport with one another—and had fun—much more than if they had been sitting passively in a classroom listening to their teacher.

What Can a Parent Do?

Let's look at some ways to bring autonomy, competence, relatedness, meaning, and joy into your teen's life—both at school and at home.

Autonomy

Autonomy is all about leaning into allowing your child to make age-appropriate choices whenever possible, aiming, as your child matures, to serve as a consultant rather than sole decision-maker or—worst-case scenario—dictator. It doesn't mean giving your teen the freedom to do whatever they want; rather, it is supporting them in making choices that are consistent with their (and your family's) values. Above all, it involves listening to and valuing your child's opinion (even if you don't agree with it) and aiming for open two-way communication. This involves trusting them to make good decisions and to live with the consequences of bad ones.

Autonomy for Your Teen as It Relates to School

We've seen how powerless kids can feel in the face of rigid school systems and societal pressure, so anything that you can do to encourage their autonomy during the school day could make a huge impact. This doesn't mean the sudden removal of your supportive involvement; rather, it is about keeping autonomy in mind as an aim. Here are some suggestions about how to work within this framework, gradually handing over control as appropriate.

- As much as possible, your teen should be in charge of tracking and completing homework assignments. It can be helpful to discuss organizational systems that work for them if they seem to struggle with this piece (and the earlier they can figure out a system the better). Stixrud and Johnson, the authors of *The Self-Driven Child,* whom I introduced you to in chapter 9, make a compelling case for not engaging in homework battles and having your child deal with the consequences when they fall behind—this is better instilled earlier when the fallout may be less extreme. For some kids, though, like Wren, who struggle with ADHD, executive dysfunction, or mental health challenges, assistance may be needed. You know your kid best, so aim for as much autonomy as they can handle, increasing it over the years, while being available to support them as necessary.

- Give your child the opportunity to fail. An extension of the previous point, your child can develop a strong sense of ownership and autonomy when you take away their safety net and they can see where their actions take them. Try this in areas where the stakes are low. For example, if you remind them to sign up for Driver Education and they don't, instead of nagging them, allow them to bear the disappointment of missing out. They'll likely figure out a way to prioritize sign-up the next time the course is offered.

- Kids can and should be in the driver's seat when choosing electives. It's one of the few places they may have a choice in classes, and if they have a say in what they learn, they're more likely to enjoy it. Marisa, a teen who was involved in social justice in her community, was excited to take an elective in government and politics. Sophomore Jake signed up for a social studies elective called Moral Dilemmas at the Movies. His parents were dubious, thinking that "sitting around talking about movies" didn't sound rigorous enough, but they decided to support their son's choice, knowing that he had a full plate of other demanding classes on his schedule. It turned out to be one of their best parenting decisions. Not only did Jake love the class, finding it both relaxing and thought-provoking, but he found a whole new group of classmates to hang out with and discovered a passion for film—he even got his family involved in monthly movie nights.

- Allow your teen to choose their own after-school activities, providing support and guidance along the way. This can be tricky, especially if you will have to provide transportation and financial support, so be prepared to discuss what will work for your family. You may have to compromise—and they may too. Perhaps high school soccer is a better choice than an all-intensive travel league, given the time commitments and your and your teen's mutual agreement to establish more balance in life.

- Encourage them to be in charge of their school and after-school schedules, including when they may need your assistance in getting to a rehearsal or a game and when they'd like your attendance. Help them learn to prioritize by talking through the stakes. Should they skip practice to go to a friend's birthday party? Perhaps, or perhaps not, but ultimately the decision and the consequences are theirs.
- Let your teen handle school-related issues and problems (why a paper is late, whether they can get an extension, clarification on homework) rather than doing so for them. But always send the message that you are there for them and available to consult if needed.
- As I discussed in chapter 8, encourage your teen to take the lead as much as they can in the college application process, while being supportive and ready to discuss their options when they'd like. It can be a difficult balance to master, as the process can feel overwhelming and emotions can get in the way. Taylor, a junior at a high-achieving school in New York State, shared how upsetting it was for her when her parents gave her a list of colleges that they thought would be a good fit for her, especially as they were all Ivy League schools—and she was hoping to go to school on the West Coast. It was hard for her to even think about making her own choices, knowing that she would be disappointing her parents from the outset.

Autonomy for Your Teen at Home

As with their school life, encouraging opportunities for autonomy at home begins with respectful communication between you and your teen.

- Acknowledge your child's perspective and validate their thoughts and experiences. Ultimately, you want to honor that they are their own person with opinions, beliefs, values, and thoughts. An unequal power dynamic will always exist in your relationship, even if it is unspoken, and it's important not to use it as unnecessary leverage. If your child challenges you on why they should do something that you have asked them to, do *everything* in your power to avoid saying, "Because I told you to." Not only would it undermine their autonomy, but it would also not inspire confidence in your rationality. One parent recounted to me his struggle with his twelve-year-old son around taking out the garbage. When the boy asked, "Why should I?" the parent, after a few exasperated missteps, came up with a good reason: "Because there are certain things that need to be done to keep our home functioning and everyone needs to pitch in."

- Offer choices. Whenever possible, start at an early age to give your child choices so that they can see that their opinion counts and that they have a say. I taught parents in my pediatric practice to avoid yes/no questions with their two-year-olds because a toddler's default answer is often no. I would use this strategy often in my own home, and I remember asking my young daughter who was resistant to wearing shoes whether she wanted to wear the black or the blue ones. When she answered no, I replied, "That wasn't one of the options." It's never too late to start giving your child choices, even if it has not been a consistent practice in the past. The key is to let them know that they have the right to exercise their choice, within a framework of possible options. As they grow older, you can broaden the choices and include what may seem like riskier options (to you) that can support their growing autonomy. Would they prefer you to pick them up from the game or to take the subway home with their friends?
- Encourage independence. You'll likely remember Kurt and Jennifer and their son Peter from chapters 8 and 9. They

allowed Peter to ride his bicycle the short distance to his friends' homes when he was eight years old. Some parents were initially shocked when he appeared at the door without a grown-up. After reaching out to Kurt and Jennifer to discuss the matter, they saw how the boy's independence had been scaffolded over time, small steps overseen by his parents leading to the granting of more freedom. Several of the other parents began to allow their kids to do the same within a framework that expected their child to take appropriate responsibility in exchange for ever-increasing independence.

- Having full responsibility for small things fosters responsibility for more and bigger things over time. A parent told me a story about her daughter who was six or seven when she became fascinated by the small hermit crabs scuttling along the beach. She scooped a dozen or so of them into a bucket so that she could study them, but her mother said that the crabs didn't seem very happy, all tumbled in together. She told her daughter that she could look after one hermit crab at a time, and that if the crab seemed content, then she could care for two or three at once. The child took her job seriously, providing sand, shade, and water to the crab, before releasing it back into the wild, at which point she was allowed to study two more crabs. She learned that she was responsible for the crab's welfare and that it meant something to be trusted with this role. There are likely many areas in your teen's life where they can exercise responsibility and grow as a person. It could be caring for a pet, making sure that their favorite snacks are on the weekly shopping list, handling a small budget, or learning to make simple meals.

- Encourage your child to think independently, form judgments, and express and defend their opinions. Help them develop a set of values that guides their lives. In the current achievement-oriented environment that constitutes childhood and adolescence, many kids have not had the chance to ponder what they might value themselves, quite apart from the achievement-related metrics that are central to their lives. We tend to ask kids what they want to be when they grow up. Perhaps the better question might be *who* they want to be and what are the values that they want to guide their lives by. In Charlie Mackesy's book *The Boy, the Mole, the Fox and the Horse,* the horse asks the boy, "What do you want to be when you grow up?" and the boy answers with one simple word, "Kind."

Competence

As a parent, you have many ways to support your child in developing a sense of competence—feeling good about their knowledge, skills, effort, and performance—in a culture that asks for perfection and often makes them feel incompetent if they fall short. You can help them see that they are capable in many spheres of their lives—even, and especially when, they may consider themselves not good enough in some areas. In the case of Wren, who was demoralized by the demands of school, it was their mom who initially bolstered their sense of competency by actively helping them find avenues for their interests and by refusing to view their struggles as in any way being their fault or an indicator of their value. Over time Wren was able to find a way—at the zoo—to build their own sense of competence.

Competence for Your Teen as It Relates to School

- Trust them to get there. For some kids, the first step toward independence is getting to school without their parents' help, and it can really boost their sense of competence as well. If your school provides a bus service or your teen can take public transportation, or walk or ride their bike, give them permission to do that rather than always giving them a ride. Mastering the ability to travel to and from school provides a sense of competence in many areas—including navigating traffic, strangers, adverse weather, and time management.

- Give your child a chance to figure out their homework. If you're like many parents, you likely feel the urge to jump in and help your child at the earliest sign of struggle with homework. In part, it's because you want to be caring and show that you're there for your kid, but over the years, as the stakes have grown higher, your eagerness to assist may be more related to concern that they'll get a bad grade if you don't. Resist that urge to help if you can! Be supportive, but first, allow them to take a stab at it themselves. This will give them the practice they need to take the lead in navigating difficulty, resolving problems, and learning to make constructive decisions for themselves.

- Counterbalance messages of incompetence. For teens caught up in achievement culture, the opportunity to feel incompetent appears to be everywhere—in school as well as in extracurriculars. There always seems to be someone achieving more than them or getting a higher score than they can hope to land. Make sure that they don't tie their sense of competence only to academics or where they might be accepted for college. Be sure to recognize them for effort, kindness, diligence, curiosity, and other qualities—the things you adore and admire in them. One teen told me how she'd overheard her parents talking with some friends one evening. The adults had been discussing their kids' various accomplishments and she'd heard her mom say, "Sarah's doing well in class too, but, you know, the other day I was on my way to work when I saw her going to school with her friends. There was an elderly woman waiting to cross the street and I saw Sarah ask if she needed help. It made me really happy to see that. And I told her so.

It's important to me that she knows that she's a good, kind member of our community."

- Let competency shine during college applications. It's to be expected that your teen may feel overwhelmed by the process—especially if you've made it into a high-stakes event—but let them know you trust that they can handle it. Imagine how they will feel if they write their own admissions essay versus how they will feel if you (largely) do it for them. Would it be a better essay if you bring your years of experience and advice to the process? Maybe. Will it be good enough—and better for your teen's individual growth—if they do it themselves? Let them know that you're there for advice or feedback, when and as needed, but they must lead the process—after all, they are the expert in where they want to go to college.
- Be supportive. What does that support look like? Help them see their strengths and where effort/hard work has helped in the past. Encourage your teen's feelings of competence (You've got this!) and—crucially—help them restructure their thoughts if they are experiencing maladaptive perfectionism or cognitive distortions like magnification or all-or-nothing thinking. You can refer back to chapters 5 and 6 to refresh your memory and find some helpful strategies.

Competence for Your Teen at Home

It's easy to fall into the trap of taking the lead on everything around the home. I certainly did. Sometimes this comes from the idea that it's simpler and faster to do things yourself. Often it can stem from seeing how much your child is handling with school and extracurricular activities and not wanting to add anything else to their plate, but in reality you're not doing them any favors. You can undermine your child's development, in terms of both skill-building and the sense of competence that comes from it. At home, make a point of looking for ways for your child to feel a sense of competence outside of their school and extracurricular activities.

- Provide opportunities to develop new skills and take on responsibilities at home. These could include doing chores, taking care of pets, playing with siblings, grocery shopping, or planning a family outing. Let your teen see how effective they can be in different activities, and take on board the message that achievement or overachievement is not the most important aim. The teen son of one of my colleagues discovered that he really liked playing with his younger cousins, especially how much they looked up to him and how his aunt and uncle were genuinely appreciative of his informal babysitting, which also freed up the couple to spend some time together, just the two of them.

- Enlist your teen's help with dinner prep and, particularly if they enjoy it, encourage them to take the lead on a new recipe. Food prep and cooking open up an endless array of ways to feel competent—from boiling an egg or whipping up pasta dishes or desserts to planning and preparing cookouts or dinner parties.

- Engage your teen in a home improvement project and praise them as they learn new skills.

- Help them develop navigation skills around your town and when traveling to a new place on vacation. Give them a chance to decipher the local metro system. One teen with an exceptional sense of direction was given the job of getting her family back to the hotel when on vacation in New York City. No matter where they were, she could be relied on to return them safely from their city wanderings. Their trust in her helped her see herself in a new light.

- Avoid micromanaging their schedule. Hovering over them or overseeing every facet of their lives sends the message that you don't think they are capable of doing it themselves—and ultimately they won't be able to if they're never given the chance to figure it out.

- Try to be mindful of how often you nag or criticize rather than praise and encourage. And beware of words like *always* and *never,* as in "You never clean up after yourself!" or "You're always late to everything." Instead, find opportunities to provide your child with unexpected positive feedback and expressions of gratitude. Thank them for their contributions to family life, particularly ones that are not on their chore list. "I appreciate you calling Grandpa yesterday. He told me how happy it made him."

- If they are struggling with a big task, help them break it down into small steps that are easier to tackle. In that way, a huge sense of incompetence—and the accompanying paralysis—can give way to multiple feelings of competence as they progress through each stage.

- Help them find after-school activities that they're good at. Like Wren's mom, you could assist in finding opportunities outside of school where they can feel competent. The focus here is on your child: What are they good at and what might they enjoy?

- Highlight their strengths. Be sure to help them see facets of themselves that are not related to achievement, or doing, and identify them as strengths. These might include humor, empathy, kindness, courage, honesty, keeping calm, or determination. "I noticed how patient you were with your sister during dinner. It would have been so much easier to get mad at her and you didn't. I think patience may be your superpower!"

Relatedness

Relatedness—feeling a sense of connection to others—is the third pillar of self determination theory, and parents can take steps to promote it in their kids' lives and thereby potentially enhance their mental health and well-being.

Relatedness For Your Teen as It Relates to School

- Encourage your child to select classes and after-school activities that have a collaborative component and aren't excessively pressured by coaches or other supervisors. These might include volunteer activities, drama or dance, orchestra, yearbook club, color guard, or some team sports. Wren identified the community of fellow animal lovers at the zoo as an important contributor to their improved mental health.
- Try to discourage excessive competitiveness with peers, as well as toxic comparison, which I described in chapter 5. If your child is doing well in school, encourage them to help their friends who are struggling with certain subjects to figure things out. Be open to your teen having friends over to study or hang out. You don't need to go to any special trouble to create a welcoming atmosphere—but try to keep it pressure-free.
- Help your child see themselves as part of a school community—that they're all in it together. Encourage them to join or set up study groups to tackle homework together. If they aren't into sports and dislike pep rallies, see if you can help them identify other groups where they feel like they could make connections. Suggest that they support friends in their after-school performances by attending the school play or dance and music concerts.

- If you have the time, energy, and inclination, join the PTA or parent booster club and show that being part of their school community is important to you.

Relatedness for Your Teen at Home

- Prioritize time for family togetherness, making clear that it is important and not expecting it to just happen organically. Put it on the schedule, just as you would volleyball practice or a piano lesson, and involve your child in setting the time. Consider making it a regular part of family life, and make it enjoyable! David and Rochelle decided to start by blocking off Saturday afternoons for family time with a technology prohibition and some active engagement whenever possible, such as nature walks, visits to a natural history museum, or just quiet time at home. The focus was on being together, which sometimes involved an activity and sometimes did not.

- Encourage your child to make time to hang out with friends—time when they can be together, unsupervised by adults. Let them know that their friends are welcome to come over to your house—as long as household rules are followed by everyone.

- Let your child know that they matter, that they are a crucial part of the family and play an important role—and not just as a student. Spend plenty of positive time with them with engaged and friendly interactions—and by all means, try to stay off your phone or laptop.

- Value family, friends, and personal connections, and model making time for other people. Paul and Linda made visits to Paul's aging father in a nursing home a weekly priority, and encouraged their two teen children to join them whenever possible. They put it on the calendar and scheduled around it and often had to turn down other options. Over the years, the kids started to automatically schedule their time around the visit too.

Meaning and Joy

Although meaning and joy are not formal parts of self-determination theory, they were essential components of the success that we achieved at SLU. They are not about doing more or achieving more; rather, they are about loving something simply in the doing of it. The SLU medical students exercised autonomy in their choices of electives and volunteer activities, and they experienced a sense of relatedness and competence in their chosen endeavors, but integral to their flourishing was the joy and meaning that infused their efforts and buoyed their spirits. These are also vitally important components of Andrea Vescelius's class. Every assignment is designed to encourage kids to find insights and meaning, and in that process to experience the simple joy of learning. As a parent, you can help guide your child toward experiencing more meaning and more joy in their life, both at home and at school, and the difference this makes could be transformational for them.

Meaning and Joy for Your Teen as They Relate to School

- Help your child see beyond the narrow focus of grades and enjoy learning for its own sake. Support them as they explore and discover a passion. Is it computers, bees, meteorology, or Taiko drumming? Encourage them to choose activities because they think they will find joy and meaning in them, not because they think it will look good on their résumé. Following a talk I gave at the California high school that Jason attended, he came up to me hesitantly with a classmate. The two boys wanted to know if robotics would be a good thing for them to be invested in learning about. I asked, "Do you love it?" Immediately, they said yes. "Then, absolutely!" I said. They broke into huge grins, gave each other a big high-five, and walked off chattering excitedly. That's what you want your child to feel in some sphere in their life, and I hoped it would make a difference in Jason's life, bringing him a glimmer of light amid the grind.

- Open up the world to them by connecting them to the bigger picture. As an experienced adult, you can help them see beyond the confines of their school-dominated lives and realize that they are part of something beyond themselves. Have them think about what and who else is out there, in other states, across the country, and around the world. How is their school powered by electricity? Where does their food come from? How would they change the way the school spends its money? Get them to think beyond what's in front of them by encouraging them to ask why? and what if?

- Consider whether a change in schools may be warranted. Christina was a freshman who loved to dance. Her public school allowed no time for electives and the homework load crowded out any time for her to pursue this passion, leaving her feeling exhausted and depressed. Her mom thought that perhaps a school for the arts might be a better fit and helped Christina explore this option, ultimately leading to her acceptance at a performing arts magnet school where she can pursue her passion and is flourishing. Sometimes the solution to a difficult situation is a different situation.

Meaning and Joy for Your Teen at Home

- Encourage them to develop and make time for personal passions big and small, whether drawing or photography, birdwatching, board games like chess, or climate change activism. Don't be dismissive of their interests or try to move them toward more "résumé-worthy" options. Let your child experiment and discover for themselves who they are and what makes them tick.

- Help them see their identities as something beyond scores, grades, goals scored, or drama production leads. Embrace Wren's mom's assertion "You are not your grades."

- Model these behaviors yourself. What gives your life meaning? When I was working at SLU, I made it clear to my daughters how much I loved my work and how it was a wonderful thing to work in a position where you regularly felt like you were making a difference in people's lives. Other people have interests outside of work too and share them with their kids. One mother developed a love of sports photography after her daughter took up skiing—and they were able to pursue their passions together.

- Help them see beyond their own self-absorption. The educational system and achievement culture are powerful forces in developing an excessive focus on self—it's too often about *my* score, *my* grades, and *my* success in college applications. Try to help your kid see that life isn't just a race, that finding things that you love and engaging with people you care about and who care about you are essential components of flourishing.

- Travel to interesting places with them. Kurt and Jennifer were able to afford a trip to Hawaii, in part because they weren't sinking large sums of money each year into private schools or club sports. While there, Peter was able to try snorkeling for the first time and he even tried jumping from a cliff over a waterfall, experiences he will likely never forget. But you don't have to travel across oceans to find fascinating places to visit—see what you might discover in your own part of the world.

- Encourage and role-model being interested in the world (the news, politics, entertainment, etc.). Talk about compelling or thought-provoking articles you've read, TV shows you've watched, or conversations you've had that piqued your interest—and that may invite your teen's curiosity.

- Try to make time for play, for them and for yourself *with* them. Play shouldn't just be for younger kids; it can be an important part of life for teens and adults alike. Play is a great way to enhance well-being, in part because it tends to include the three pillars of self-determination theory. It involves choice in what to play at, relatedness as you engage in play collaboratively, and competence when play goes well. Well-being is not the only potential benefit: It can promote a sense of balance in life, support creativity and problem-solving, and deepen relationships with others. I believe that many kids and families today have a play deficit that should be addressed and rectified. Play can take many forms—sports or physical activity such as hiking, dancing, frisbee, or tossing a baseball; video or board games; improv games such as charades; crossword puzzles and word games; or creative play such as painting, journaling, making short videos, building something, baking, or working on a garden project together. The possibilities are endless.

Shifting your parenting approach to more fully encouraging autonomy, competence, and relatedness in school, extracurricular activities, and at home, along with embracing meaning and joy, can counteract the negative effects experienced by many teens as they jump through the endless hoops of school and achievement culture. You're likely to see more engagement and more curiosity in your child, and the development of broader, richer, and more fulfilling goals both in their current life and in their hoped-for future. They will have more opportunities to foster a sense of self that is fuller and more complex than striving to be a perfect student. They'll begin to embrace the message that there is not a single path to success, but many—and that success itself can take many different shapes and forms. They will—I hope—be able to look back on their teen years with more pleasure and satisfaction than if they—and you—had fallen into the trap of accepting that the cost of success was an inevitable, interminable grind. As you navigate achievement culture, keep in mind that you're trying to raise a well-rounded, compassionate individual with unique strengths and an enthusiasm for life that will carry into their adult years—not a success-bot whose only metric of achievement is their GPA and test scores. Remember that combatting unnecessary stress, relentless pressure, and maladaptive perfectionism is a good fight, and that a childhood that abounds with meaning and joy is one worth striving for.

Conclusion

As I reach the end of writing this book, let me pause to reflect on the truths I have tried to bring forward about the pressured lives of kids in school settings, which, I believe, are among the primary contributors to the current youth mental health crisis in this country. I hope that many of you who recognize aspects of your child's experience in the situations I've described will take heart from understanding that the problem does not lie with your child but with a system and culture that have spun out of control. I also hope that my words will sound an alarm that will spur action on a number of fronts. These include enacting ways to help your kid enjoy a more balanced life and develop a resilient identity in the face of stress, and sparking change at schools and in the sphere of extracurricular activities. Sometimes this involves advocating for less, not more—less homework, less time spent in after-school endeavors or on crazy travel schedules for club sports, fewer late-night study sessions and early morning practices. I believe that creating space in a young person's life is more important than stuffing it to the bursting point with "enrichment" opportunities and activities undertaken for the purpose of showcasing accomplishments in college applications.

I have offered tools to help your teen better manage the problematic mindsets and distorted thinking patterns that make the distress that so many feel even worse. I've provided lenses that you can use in your and your child's consideration of choices related to schools, coursework, extracurricular activities, and the college application process. I've tried to demonstrate how self-determination theory can inform and guide you in creating a safe, supportive, nurturing environment at home—one that nourishes your child, rather than adding to the pressure they are already enduring. And for those who have the time, inclination, and desire, I've created an advocacy road map for how to lead much-needed efforts for systemic changes in schools. (This can be found in the Supplemental Resources at the end of this book.)

But, perhaps most important, I've given you scientific evidence that backs up what you've been likely feeling for so long: that achievement culture is harming our kids, that we shouldn't be sacrificing our kids' mental health for the singular goal of gaining admission to an elite or highly selective college, and that excessive focus on this brand of success is ultimately a dangerous trap. At the core of this book is my strong belief that we need to prioritize our kids' mental health in the face of a widely accepted and false idea that intensive school-related pressure will help them succeed in life. I believe this notion is wrongheaded and that it threatens instead to undermine a child's best chances of flourishing.

Advocating for balance in a child's life should be seen as sensible, natural, and something we owe our children. The tides have turned so dramatically, however, toward overscheduling and ratcheting up demands that it requires a great resolve, and some courage, to face and deal with an irony that is hiding in plain sight: The narrow, cutthroat path to "success" is driving an overwhelming number of teens into depression, anxiety, and, in some cases, despair. There is no sole culprit: it isn't just about screen time, or social media, or club sports, or too much homework, or academic metrics, or compromised family life. Rather, the pile-up of all these factors is leaching the joy out of life for too many teens. But as you've seen, there are solutions, and many situations that look quite dire can be improved and fixed. My hope is that, along with data and research, I've given you the confidence you need to make different choices. To have the courage to say no to unwarranted, unprecedented pressure and, moreover, to feel good about doing so because you're putting your child's mental health first—and that is no small thing.

Already I've seen some parents and kids making choices to extricate themselves from the snares and take back their lives, and many of them have described to me their hope and satisfaction in the changes they've made. While it hasn't been easy, they saw their choices as clear and many of them are thriving. Emma's parents ultimately decided to pull her out of her high-pressure school, despite her protests, and enroll her in an online learning platform. They decided that they could no longer bear to see their daughter struggle so much—it just wasn't worth it. Her tics have disappeared, and her anxiety has diminished. She misses playing volleyball, but she is so much happier now. She and her parents are looking at other schools in their town that might be a better fit and where she could potentially enroll next year. They know now what they didn't know before—that academic rigor must come in a different package for Emma.

Olivia is now in fifth grade and is still involved in soccer. Her parents don't see a better alternative because all of her friends are on the team. They believe that pulling her out of the sport would likely mean she would have no one to hang out with after school and that she would turn to screens for entertainment. Olivia's parents are familiar with maladaptive perfectionism and the way it impacts her life and are using cognitive restructuring to help her. Already they are seeing positive results. Olivia's meltdowns are less frequent and less intense, and she seems less anxious overall, which has led to reduced stress for the entire family.

Brett's entreaties to Duke admissions did not lead to his acceptance there, but he managed to complete his other applications to a wide range of colleges, and he landed in another excellent school. He has jumped into his freshman year and is having a blast. His experience has led him to realize that chasing a singular goal was misguided in many ways. He has embraced a new approach to his studies and extracurricular pursuits, looking for fulfillment, engagement, connection, meaning, and enjoyment.

Katherine, the medical student who struggled with maladaptive perfectionism and impostor phenomenon, is now thriving as a clinical faculty member in ophthalmology. She still uses cognitive restructuring techniques as necessary, and she attempts to balance her long work hours with activities that bring her joy—time with loved ones, time enjoying nature, and, especially important to her, plenty of sleep. She knows the importance of prioritizing her mental health.

As I travel the country, I hear from an increasing number of parents who, like Kurt and Jennifer, are saying no to the pressure, choosing a less demanding and stressful path for their children and themselves, and seeing early dividends from it. I also hear from other families who are still caught up in the culture of high-achieving schools but who are doing what they can to temper the effects of it. They're creating low-pressure zones at home and encouraging their teens to cut back on extracurriculars, broaden their college search to include options beyond the usual list of elites, and think about what they're really looking for in a college experience rather than chasing other people's definitions of success. And these small changes are making a difference.

I'm hopeful that as more parents escape the success trap, or knowingly evade it, the movement toward prioritizing our children's mental health and well-being will ripple outward and it will become the norm—that one day soon we'll look back and wonder how we could ever have done anything else.

Supplemental Resources

Fundamental change is desperately needed in our education system along with strong parent advocates for reform, as the system is unlikely to change unless pressure is applied. However, many parents are stretched too thin already and don't have the time or energy to lead the charge. This supplemental section is primarily for those who are interested in taking on a leadership role, but I hope you read through regardless—and that you find yourself inspired!

Advocating for Change: We Need a Revolution!

I once spoke with lifelong educator Jim Mahoney, who served as a school district superintendent for fifteen years, about why schools were so slow to change even in the face of compelling evidence that they should. I shared with him my perception that they were unlikely to modify the way learning happens *unless parents demand it.* He answered immediately and emphatically, "Absolutely!" Schools, he explained, are largely a reflection of what a community wants and thinks (though state accountability systems also contribute), and the status quo is maintained because the pain (and personal threat) of staying the same is less than that of changing. In other words, unless a school is compelled to change because of significant parental, or societal, action and pressure, it is easier and safer for them to keep going as they are. We know there is a teen mental health crisis in this country, and, as I've demonstrated throughout the book, some of the biggest drivers of poor mental health outcomes in kids and teens exist in our schools. It's time that parents demand that schools change and put student well-being first.

As we've seen, parents can make great progress in improving teens' mental health at the individual level through making changes at home and in the extracurricular sphere. We can effect these changes through the following:

- Acknowledging the role of academic pressure and achievement culture in the increase in anxiety and depression in teens
- Reducing unnecessary pressure at home
- Recognizing and better managing problematic mindsets and cognitive distortions
- Helping kids develop broader goals and create more complex identities
- Reducing extracurricular overload to free up time for deep connection as a family
- Finding ways for kids to feel competent
- Ensuring that teens experience a sense of belonging
- Giving kids more autonomy in their lives outside of school and helping them find activities that bring them real meaning and joy

Doing some or all of the above can make a critical difference in your teen's life—the difference, in some cases, between sound and poor mental well-being. However, much lies beyond the direct control of individual parents. This supplement addresses how to use your collective voices as parents (and teens as well) to push for action in bringing change to schools. It draws on my success at implementing significant changes at SLU, the lessons I learned from my failure to effect change at my daughter's high school, and my research and discussions over the years with parents, students, teachers, and schools. I'll provide you with key components and strategies to mount an effective change campaign.

My experience at SLU taught me several crucial factors about change. First, change is possible, so keep going no matter the obstacles. Second, bringing about change needs to be approached in the right way—taking the time to think things through is vital as you'll likely be dealing with entrenched systems and mindsets. Third, be aware that relatively simple changes can produce huge positive results—so don't be tempted to overcomplicate matters or become caught up in the notion that significant change needs to be grand and sweeping. The core changes that we enacted at SLU—reducing class time by 10 percent, cutting the amount of information we were teaching, freeing up time for electives, and changing our grading system—cost almost nothing in terms of financial resources and little in the way of faculty effort, for trimming content is not the same as an overhaul of the curriculum or a radical change in how we taught. Yet these simple changes led to a huge reduction in student anxiety and depression rates and an increase in their overall flourishing.

I also learned that change can be dangerous for those who lead it. Ultimately, I lost my job at SLU, primarily, I'm convinced, because of the part I played in effecting change. Six years into our movement for improved mental health, we had a site visit from the body that accredits medical schools. We had sailed through this accreditation process eight years before, and I had no great worries about how we would fare. We had outstanding academic outcomes, students were enormously satisfied, and we had made numerous changes to the curriculum in a school that had not been particularly known for innovation. We were receiving national and international attention for our unprecedented success in improving medical student mental health.

Yet as soon as the site visit team arrived, we sensed trouble. They seemed to be searching for problems, and their tone was diametrically opposite to that of the previous site visitors. A few weeks later, our dean received the initial report: nineteen citations. He acted immediately, asserting in a letter to the accreditors that at least half of them were erroneous, but he was informed that he could not appeal until the full accreditation committee had reviewed the report and rendered their final decision. During that hiatus he retired, and a new dean took his place and soon received the decision that the school was being placed on probation. He chose not to appeal, despite there being numerous grounds on which to do so, and hid the notification from the accreditation committee from me until fifteen minutes before SLU's probation was headline news in the local paper. A month later he relieved me of my duties as curricular dean. There was an outpouring of support from students—a petition with six hundred signatures and a large protest, which I appreciated, but that did not change the outcome of my dismissal.[1]

This was a challenging and difficult period in my life, but I used many of the tools that I had taught the medical students to make my way through it. I took steps to maintain positive emotions and optimism. I noticed that when I worried that I would never be able to get another job that I was engaging in fortune-telling—and I disputed my thoughts. I ramped up my self-care activities, increasing the time that I exercised. Ultimately, my dismissal turned out to be the biggest professional gift of my life. I was hired by the Accreditation Council for Graduate Medical Education, initially as a senior scholar for well-being and later as vice president for well-being, giving me a tremendous platform to work on the problem of resident and faculty mental health and well-being, as well as the time and freedom to expand my research efforts in adolescent mental health and, ultimately, to write this book.

How to Bring About Change

The process of effecting change in schools can be better understood through field theory,[2] which was developed in the 1940s by Kurt Lewin, an organizational psychologist. Lewin believed that all situations exist in a state of "dynamic equilibrium" regulated by restraining and driving forces. If we view schools across this country through this lens, we could say that the driving forces—those parents wanting change—are not exceeding the restraining forces—those wanting things to stay the way they are—so, as Jim Mahoney said, it is safer for school administrators to maintain the status quo than to initiate change. In chapter 3, when student Emma was struggling with her mental health, her parents met with the head of her school. When they pleaded to reduce homework loads, the head countered that she had parents coming into her office to demand *more homework*! In simple terms, Emma's parents were outnumbered—and the amount of homework remained unchanged. Had they banded together with other concerned parents, they might have been able to increase the driving forces and, also perhaps, to sway some of the parents in the restraining forces camp by helping them understand the dangers of the status quo.

Understanding Lewin's theory of driving and restraining forces is a good place to start your activism. There are, in addition, other key elements to an effective change campaign.

Arm yourself with evidence and data. At SLU, it was critically important to bring evidence to the discussion—my plan would have been a nonstarter without it. Citing studies at three medical schools that showed no negative impacts on student academic performance, or on success in matching to residency programs, as a result of the change to pass/fail grading was essential in countering early resistance from faculty and students. In addition, bringing the alarmingly high student depression and anxiety rates to our curricular committee deliberations was, I believe, critical in accomplishing change. Had I not had that data, and had I simply reported to this committee my concern about how stressed our students were, I seriously doubt that any significant action would have been taken.

No matter what issue you are bringing to school administrators, you'll want to have a foundation of solid data to support your concerns. Hard evidence is vitally important to many people (including me). To that end, I have established a website (drstuartslavin.com) that provides key evidence about subjects such as teen mental health, sleep science, and homework recommendations that you can share with other parents and family members and bring to meetings with school administration or to school board meetings. You can also find there information about the mental health survey that I used in the eighteen schools that I studied. All of the instruments are nonproprietary, so are free to use.

Align yourself with the school's mission and values. As I shared in chapter 4, the mission statement at SLU School of Medicine included the words "education of the whole person—mind, body, spirit, and heart," and I leaned on that heavily in my campaign for change, stating that our educational approaches were not consistent with our mission statement. Look at your school's mission statement or statement of values. Are the educational approaches and outcomes consistent with those statements? Also, keep watch for statements from the school administration such as "Student mental health is our number one priority." If student mental health is poor at the school and preventive mental health actions are not being taken, you can point out the discrepancy.

Enlist allies. There is power in numbers, and I recommend that you talk to other parents to see if they are concerned about your specific issue or more general issues. You could start with the parents you know, and you could attend school events or join the PTA or school booster club to expand your network, engaging other parents in informal discussion. Once you start talking with other people, you may be surprised by the number who are equally concerned—but have said nothing because they thought it was a problem centered on their child or that change was unlikely to happen. In many cases, you will discover shared worries and gratitude for bringing up issues that are affecting many kids, parents, and families, and some fellow parents may wish to join forces with you. At that point, you can create a strategy for bringing your case to the school. If, on the other hand, you cannot find any allies, you may start to question whether your concerns and expectations are aligned with the greater school community; in this case, you may wonder whether this school is the right place for your child. As sobering a conclusion as that may be, it may be the right one.

At my daughter's school, I made a critical mistake of trying to go at it alone, lobbying the board under a naive assumption that they would hear me out as a pediatrician bearing reams of evidence and would approve the changes I recommended. Had I been aware of Lewin's theory at that time, I would have recognized that my sole voice was not sufficient as a driver for change. I should have focused more of my initial efforts on enlisting other parents. In retrospect, they were available. At an orientation for parents of tenth graders at the beginning of the academic year, I asked if there had been a change to the homework policy. When the head of school said no, there hadn't been, the room of parents erupted in groans and howls of protest. If we had banded together and organized, I think the driving forces would have been strong enough for the administration to make a change.

Here is another sobering thought: One might think that students would be strong allies in pushing for change, given the state of their lives at school, but that may not be the case. You may recall that a good portion of SLU students opposed pass/fail before they were given a strong rationale for the change. In a survey conducted by Learning InspirED, students who were more successful in school were less likely to endorse changes for more student autonomy and less teacher control in classes.[3] I believe a likely explanation is that there is some comfort in the status quo, as the rules (do what the teacher wants and you will succeed) and the rewards are clear. Another factor may be that those who are winning the competitive academic race feel that the status quo is working in their favor—even if the proposed changes may produce a better, more enjoyable, less pressured learning environment for them as well.

If possible, recruit allies with expertise in healthcare such as pediatricians, family and internal medicine physicians, adolescent medicine specialists, nurse practitioners, psychiatrists, psychologists, and other mental health providers. Their voices can be a powerful addition, particularly if they are members of your local school community.

Lower academic performance is not an acceptable outcome. While it may seem strange that school administrators are willing to accept high rates of anxiety and depression in their schools but not lower academic performance, this is the reality that we live in—so you'll have to work within this framework. You'll need to ensure that your proposed changes will not affect academic standards—the school's bottom line. At SLU, a number of faculty pushed back on my suggested changes, claiming that they would inevitably lead to poorer academic outcomes and would constitute a lowering of academic standards. I countered by saying that I did not believe that this would occur but that if it did we would reverse the changes. That effectively disarmed a potentially strong counterargument to our proposed curricular changes. I have to add that I believe academic standards are unlikely to fall, but if they do as stress falls and mental health improves, many parents may say that the change was worth it and those who want the old way will need to muster sufficient driving forces to change it back.

Raise awareness. My strong sense, based on dozens of discussions I've had over the years with educators and parents, is that the number of parents who strongly support high academic demands and pressure, and who adamantly oppose any suggestion that change could promote much-needed well-being for teens, are relatively few in number. In some communities, they constitute perhaps 10 percent or fewer. Far more parents recognize that their kids' lives (and, by extension, their own) are overly pressured and stressful; however, they are resigned to the notion that there is no other choice, seeing stress-filled lives as simply the price you pay for being able to compete these days, in school and beyond.

Among the forces that affect equilibrium, the small vocal group is the primary restraining force. The larger group who reluctantly support the status quo have much less impact as they tend to be quiet, not pushing to alter the equilibrium, unpleasant as it may be. Yet this larger group has the potential to be an important driving force; they just need to be convinced. How you raise awareness among these parents, as well as the greater school community, that the learning environment can and should be improved is a serious question that requires careful consideration and planning.

Mounting a campaign to increase public awareness sounds daunting, and it is. But without this awareness there is little chance of driving change, and some type of formal or informal organization or task force is likely to be necessary for creating a unified message and concerted effort to drive change.

Pick your battles. Don't try to change everything at once. While it may seem as if everything is wrong with your child's school, it's unrealistic to expect that wholescale change will happen. Choose one cause that matters to you and will really make a difference, and stick to it. It could be advocating for less homework or for more electives, or something else affecting your particular school community. But be clear and specific in your demands, rather than overbroad and vague. There were many other changes I could have tried for at SLU, but we kept our asks limited to what we could reasonably implement. One approach to deciding what to push for first is a prioritization tool called the impact-effort (or impact-feasibility) matrix. It puts actions or initiatives into four possible quadrants based on their potential impact and likely effort/feasibility to determine what to tackle first when considering possible initiatives. Early on in your campaign, you will want to target changes that are high impact/low effort to create momentum for further change. These are often referred to as low-hanging fruit. In some ways our change at SLU to cut class time and course content was high impact and low effort. While there were political challenges in getting this approved, the faculty effort to implement wasn't great. They didn't need to change their teaching approaches or bring in new material; they simply needed to teach less.

Push initially for changes that require little financial cost. Many schools are under intense financial pressure, so seeking initial changes that are low cost can render them more likely to be accepted. The total cost for the changes enacted at SLU was about $3,000 a year—and most of that was for food at meetings.

Don't push for change in what content is taught, just the amount of it. It's useful to keep in mind how "the other side" will receive your proposals for change, what is important to them, and, based on that, what it makes most sense to ask for. At SLU, I didn't battle with faculty about *what* they taught because I knew how invested many of them were in the content of their courses—after all, they were experts in their field and, for the most part, cared deeply about their subject matter. Instead, we created mandates on how much they taught, largely respecting their autonomy to decide the content of their lectures and courses. Creating policies that limit the amount of homework fits into this category.

Know that change is possible. Activism can be time and energy intensive, and often even demoralizing, as setbacks occur and change can be slow to happen. At times when you're feeling down or questioning your impact, it can be a valuable exercise to remind yourself that change is possible. Parents have mounted successful campaigns in the past. One example is later school start times, an evidence-based accommodation that supports adolescent learning, which I will return to later in this section. In 2014 in Fairfax, Virginia, a local advocacy group composed mostly of parents pushed for and eventually succeeded in getting high school start times changed from 7:30 a.m. to between 8:00 and 8:10 a.m.[4] Soon thereafter, Seattle Public Schools followed suit, changing high school start times to 8:45 a.m.[5] Over the years, implementing later start times has become a national movement, with significant changes taking place in more than forty-six states. Local groups have been supported by organizations such as Start School Later, which comprises an international coalition of more than 165 volunteer-led chapters that bring awareness to the need for more sleep and advocate for change in school policies and state laws relating to start times. You can also look for strategies from other successful school campaigns, such as book banning—even if you don't align with their goals. The idea is to see what works and what you can learn and bring to your own campaign.

Consider joining or running for school board. If you have the time and the inclination and your child is in a public school, consider running for school board. It is an effective way to get involved and have a direct say in the running of your local school. Especially in smaller districts, it tends not to be terribly expensive to mount a campaign, though it can be time consuming. If your child is in a private school, see if you can work your way into being selected to serve on the board. I was able to do that by developing a relationship with the head of school at my daughter's school.

Watch out for potential barriers. Change can be slow and halting, so be prepared that you likely won't see quick results. Any change to the status quo will be perceived as risky by administrators, teachers, parents, and students who cling to an outdated notion of how "rigor" is upheld and preserved and believe that academic success can only be achieved through traditional methods. You will encounter a variety of mistaken assertions intended to block change, and you need to be ready to counter them.

- "Kids need to be pushed academically—it's a competitive world out there." You can counter that the constant push for more in terms of grades and achievement does not result in excellence. There is a breaking point—and the teen mental health crisis would suggest we have reached it.
- "Depression and anxiety are individual issues; they aren't caused by the environment." This is a common misunderstanding, and one that data can disprove. You can provide research that links academic pressure to mental health conditions in teens—the studies that show suicides and suicide attempts peaking during school months (and decreasing during vacations) are especially striking. The most effective counter, however, is getting data from your specific school through surveys to measure depression and anxiety. If a majority of kids are found to suffer from depression and/or anxiety, it is hard to make the case that this problem is limited to a few and is just an individual problem.
- "But my kids are doing fine." Many parents will say that their kids are doing well in the current system. And maybe they are—or maybe they are being Stanford Ducks. Either way, you can counter by saying that this may be true, but many kids are not doing fine, and the school's mandate is to serve all students. Also, there's no evidence that the kids who are thriving wouldn't "do fine" if changes were made to reduce demands and

pressure. Academic performance at SLU didn't fall when we cut back on things; it improved—meaning that everyone benefited, even those without depression or anxiety in the first place.

- "Social media and smartphones are the problem, not school." I am not arguing that social media and smartphones are not a problem—I believe that they are a challenge for parents and students alike. My stance is that they are not the *only* problem and that a hyperfocus on them as the cause of teen mental health problems hides other reasons—including academic pressure and achievement culture in schools. Bring forward evidence from this book, its associated website, and other sources to counter this argument.

What to Campaign For

As I described in chapter 8, many schools need serious reform, but it is not possible for everything to be changed, especially not all at once. I would recommend using the impact-feasibility matrix to sequence your push for changes in the following manner. This is not a strict guideline, however. You can move some initiatives forward on the list if you think they are warranted and can combine them if you think that makes sense. For example, reducing homework loads and changing to block schedules could be advocated for at the same time.

Survey Students

I believe that having data about depression and anxiety rates, sleep, amount of homework, and perceptions of stressors in your local high school from the outset can be of great value. Surveys for this data can be a powerful tool to push for change, as they were for me at SLU. They can also, if repeated yearly or every other year, help track whether changes are making a positive difference. We desperately need schools to make these changes and demonstrate, as I did at SLU, that they can lead to improvements to mental health without compromising academic performance at all. These surveys should be anonymous and careful protocols for student safety should be followed. Unlike the mental health screening that is being done in some schools, which is typically used to identify kids with mental health problems so that they can be referred for care, they are not generally used to assess mental illness rates in the students overall. The instruments I used and suggested guidance for adminstration are available on my website.

Reduce Homework Loads

Try to get your school to implement the guidelines we described in chapter 8, namely the "ten-minute rule," so that ninth graders should get no more than ninety minutes per weeknight and twelfth graders should get no more than two hours. Don't settle for thirty minutes per class per night if the school day includes six or seven periods. Ask that teachers coordinate with one another and remain aware of deadlines on big projects for other classes, as well as school play performances or sports championships that are likely to affect students' schedules.

Open a discussion about homework policies for weekends and consider pushing for a policy that limits or prohibits homework over holiday breaks. Some schools have homework bans over all vacations, including long weekends, allowing students to relax, recover, and enjoy time with family and friends. Push to limit, or prohibit entirely, deadlines for long-term projects soon after returns from breaks, as many students often spend their breaks mired in these projects. Be aware that instituting policies is an important first step but that it will likely not be sufficient. The policies *must* be accompanied by a commitment and concrete plan to monitor homework levels and intervene with individual teachers who are exceeding the limits. Remember to bring data and allies on your mission.

Shift to Block Schedules

Block scheduling is the most common scheduling innovation. It has the potential to reduce demands and pressure on students, and although research evidence supporting its efficacy remains limited, it seems logical that four classes per day instead of six, seven, or even eight, could lead to decreased homework loads and reduce the likelihood and intensity of multiple assignments coming due or numerous exams occurring on a single day. I've found in conversations with teens who have experienced both traditional and block schedules that they uniformly prefer blocks. They find that blocks make it easier to juggle and handle the quantity of schoolwork and that longer classes allow for more depth in teaching and a less frenzied feeling.

Increase Elective Time

As we've seen, kids can have a chance to flourish when they are able to make their own choices, and increasing elective time expands opportunities for them to feel some sense of autonomy and meaning. A sophomore student who loved drawing and painting was miserable in a school with a traditional schedule, no elective time, and a huge homework load that crowded out time for her to pursue this passion outside of school. She was accepted to an arts-focused boarding school where core classes are largely restricted to morning hours, freeing up the afternoon for her to dedicate to visual arts. She is thriving with the change now that she has an outlet for her creativity. There are many ways for both public and private schools to bring in electives and free time for students to pursue learning and other activities that really interest them, and it can be a relatively easy option for schools to introduce.

Move to Later School Start Times

Kyla Wahlstrom, a researcher at the University of Minnesota, has demonstrated the enormous benefits of starting school later for high schoolers, including increased sleep duration, improved academic performance, better attendance and lower tardiness rates, less daytime sleepiness, reduced symptoms of depression, and fewer teen car accidents.[6] As a result of her and others' work, many schools have adopted "late starts," where the school day commences at 8:30 a.m. or 9:00 a.m., rather than between 7:30 a.m. and 8:00 a.m., which is the norm, or even, alarmingly, 7:00 a.m. This is a great step, allowing a little extra sleep time for many students (depending on the relative flexibility of their family's morning schedule), but there are many more schools where these rules have yet to be implemented.

As mentioned earlier in the chapter, other parents have had success in advocating collectively for later school start times. I recommend finding like-minded parents and perhaps partnering with an organization like Start Schools Later, which has considerable expertise in this area, and then taking research to the school's administration and the school board. Be prepared to dig in—the evidence is on your side, but you're dealing with a systemic resistance to change.

Get Teachers and Coaches on the Same Schedule

Another intervention for parents to strive for is greater coordination among teachers, coaches, drama directors, and so on, helping them stay informed and mindful about when academic demands are peaking. Parents are the ones who see the whole picture of both academic demands and extracurriculars and the impacts on their teens, whereas teachers and after-school coaches and theater or dance departments often operate in silos. With effective coordination, the length of practices or rehearsals can be limited or the quantity scaled back during test periods or exams. Balance is key in attaining, and maintaining, conditions that support healthy sleep—which should be a given in any kid's life, not something that feels perpetually out of reach.

Increase Self-Directed, Student-Centered, and Active Learning

This change is somewhat more difficult to adopt because it requires teachers to change *how* they teach and often requires resources to engage external consultants to help with the change. While parent groups can advocate for this new teaching approach, school administrators will likely be the ones exploring which organizations to enlist in facilitating its implementation.

Provide More Mental Health Support and Tools

While our aim is to get schools to address harmful elements of the environment that contribute to teen anxiety and depression, the availability of mental health and wellness resources in schools is important too. Many schools are moving to provide more in this area by offering students tools and information to bolster their mental health. One of the most robust efforts that I've seen is a collaboration between two nonprofits in Ohio—MindPeace and 1N5—which joined forces with Cincinnati Children's Hospital to promote mental health awareness and provide mental health resources and interventions. They were my partners in my surveys of students in schools in Ohio.

MindPeace has worked with public and private schools and community partners to develop and maintain a network of mental health providers for children and adolescents. They work with individual schools to figure out their unique mental health needs as a population and then choose partners from the local community to provide high-quality, affordable school-based therapy services for students in need. They have also supported the creation of MindPeace rooms where kids who are struggling to control their emotions can relax and decompress, but also, most importantly, learn valuable skills to self-regulate their bodies and emotions—which they can use in the future. 1N5's mission is to prevent suicide by erasing the stigma of mental illness and advocating for optimal mental wellness. It promotes and provides educational programs such as Sources of Strength; Signs of Suicide; a speaker series; and, with Cincinnati Children's Hospital, a Youth Council for Suicide Prevention. These efforts appear to be making a difference, with surveys indicating a fall in depression and anxiety rates in these schools. There are a multitude of options to support mental health that parents can advocate for, including the introduction of teaching on self-regulation or cognitive restructuring.

Implement Changes in Grading Systems

Innovations in grading at the school or district level remain relatively rare, in large part because of the continued need for and reliance on letter or numerical grades for colleges to assess applicants. Some high schools have moved to eliminate letter grades, instead using "competency-based" or "standards-based" evaluations. This approach appears to be much more common in elite private schools, where confidence in their reputation in college admissions gives them more freedom to abandon traditional grades than public schools might have. Another policy, optional testing, is also offered in a relatively small number of schools, again most of them private. I would love to see innovation in grading spread widely, but the restraining forces will be difficult to overcome, which is why I've placed this one last in the list of change points to focus on.

We Can Do This!

Change is needed in our schools, and I firmly believe that if we join together it is possible. I hope that this book, this resource section, and the accompanying website can be important tools in this effort. We can push back against achievement culture and unnecessary academic pressure to ensure that our kids thrive. Good luck in your advocacy endeavors! Together, we can make real change happen.

Acknowledgments

In many ways, the writing of this book feels like the culmination of a personal and professional journey that began decades ago. So many of the experiences and relationships I have had over the years have woven together in unexpected ways, informing my views on adolescent mental health, an area of long-standing interest. From my personal life, I begin with my daughters and my former wife. My daughters, Alana and Natasha, showed so much grace and strength in their navigation of the pressures and demands of school and life. Their mother, Helene, was—and remains—a true force, a fierce and loving advocate for their well-being.

In my time as a pediatrician at UCLA, I am grateful for the relationships I had with so many. First, Nancy Brill, who was a great model for compassionate leadership. William F. Friedman, chair of pediatrics, believed in my potential and accorded me both time and funding for my pursuit of a master's degree in education. I learned from Michael Wilkes, co-architect of the Doctoring program, how to get things done. Brenda Hanning, Bill Heath, and Ellen Potter, administrators in pediatric education, helped me build and refine an acclaimed residency training program.

My enrollment in the MEd program at the University of Southern

California was critical to my development as an educator and researcher, and my work studying adolescent mental health would not have been possible without this training. I thank all of the faculty and my fellow students in the program, with special thanks to Steven Abrahamson, who was the epitome of what a teacher should be, and to Julie Nyquist, who taught me everything I would need to know about evaluation in research.

At Saint Louis University, I thank Greg Smith and Jim Swierkosz of the Student Affairs Office, who were wonderful partners in creating a supportive and nurturing educational environment for our students. I am indebted to my research team, John Chibnall and Deb Schindler, who were essential in assessing the impact of the changes we made at SLU. I am deeply grateful to Ginny Fendell, a clinical social worker who was instrumental in the design of our resilience curriculum and who taught me so much about cognitive restructuring. Huge thanks go to the entire staff in the Office of Curricular Affairs, led by Denise Parker, who oversaw the implementation of many of our educational reforms. Thanks also to Patricia Monteleone and Philip Alderson, deans of the medical school who were strong supporters of my work there. It was at SLU that I first began my teen mental health research, and I am very grateful to Vicki Abeles, a trailblazing documentary filmmaker and author, for forging the initial connections I had with high schools in California and encouraging me in my work.

At the Accreditation Council for Graduate Medical Education (ACGME), CEO Thomas Nasca granted me precious time to continue my work in adolescent health, and this was critical to advancing this project. I'm also grateful to my colleagues in well-being at ACGME, Nick Yaghmour and Bethanie Alden, as well as board members Josepha Cheong and Jayne Ward, for their support. Special thanks to Timothy Brigham, chief of education, for always keeping our well-being efforts for residents and faculty on a productive course. I would also like to thank Dewitt C. "Bud" Baldwin and Fred Hafferty, who served as guides and mentors in my well being work, as well as Erick French and Ken Ludmerer who offered me encouragement and guidance in recent years. I gratefully acknowledge Susan Shelton and Nancy Miller, my research partners in my studies of Ohio high schools, who are directors of two superb mental health nonprofits. In addition, Michael Sorter, director of child and adolescent psychiatry at Cincinnati Children's Hospital, and Tawni Hoeglund, a statistician extraordinaire, were instrumental in this research. Warm thanks as well to my research partners Asmira Alagic and Liz Pfau for their work on our study of college students.

Self-determination theory helped to inform my views of the steps we need to take to help youth in this country. I am immensely grateful to William R. Stixrud, Ned Johnson, and Mike Nicholson, who welcomed me into the world of SDT in K–12 education and parenting, and to Gregory Guldner and Adam Neufeld, who expanded my understanding of its connection to well-being. Very special thanks to Jason Siegel, who shared with me his goal disruption theory and gave me permission to include a chapter about it in this book.

I would like to thank, from the bottom of my heart, the students, parents, and educators who shared their personal stories, which were critical in helping me understand the pervasiveness and severity of the current youth mental health crisis in this country—how it's experienced by kids, parents, and families, as well as by the educators and mental health professionals who try to combat it so valiantly. Many of their stories are included in this book. To the SLU medical students, also my heartfelt thanks. I spearheaded changes at SLU, and you were the ones who brought them to life. There is not enough space here to name all who deserve mention, but let me call out a few: Katherine Hu, Alex Bodkin, Neil Shaw, Anu Gorakanti, Jessie Whitfield; many thanks to each one of you!

Finally, I would like to give special thanks to the small group that encouraged and collaborated with me in the long sprint to produce this manuscript. First, to Bill Stixrud, who offered strong and persistent encouragement for me to write a book proposal for an idea that had been percolating in my head for several years. Bill connected me to the best agent I could ever imagine, Jenna Land Free. Jenna was an early, critical force in shaping the form of *The Success Trap,* and she made the book proposal phase a joyful and creative experience. Jenna connected me to my partner in writing, the remarkable Lindsey Tate. Not only was she superb with the technical aspects of writing and structuring a book, but her extensive knowledge related to mental health and stress helped inform the content. Lindsey, you were an absolute joy to work with! Thanks also go to my daughter Alana, a psychiatrist, who reviewed the depression and anxiety chapters and gave me helpful feedback on both. I am immensely grateful to Thea Diklich-Newell, my editor at Ten Speed Press, for believing in this project and, as it materialized, offering insightful editorial feedback that has strengthened and enriched this book. A special thank you as well to Kristin Casemore, Emily Hotaling, Ashley Pierce, Amani Shakrah, Emma Campion, Isabelle Gioffredi, Dan Bejar, and everyone on the Ten Speed team. Finally, tremendous thanks to my partner, Noriko Gamblin, who has been an invaluable thought partner and who supported me in countless ways in what has been, perhaps, the most challenging and meaningful professional endeavor of my life as a physician and medical educator.

Notes

Introduction

1. Substance Abuse and Mental Health Services Administration (SAMHSA), *Highlights for the 2023 National Survey on Drug Use and Health* (SAMHSA, 2023), https://www.samhsa.gov/data/sites/default/files/NSDUH%202023%20Annual%20Release/2023-nsduh-main-highlights.pdf.
2. Health Resources and Services Administration, *National Survey of Children's Health: Adolescent Mental and Behavioral Health,* Data Brief (U.S. Department of Health and Human Services, 2024), https://mchb.hrsa.gov/sites/default/files/mchb/data-research/nsch-data-brief-adolescent-mental-behavioral-health-2023.pdf.
3. S. S. Luthar and S. J. Latendresse, "Children of the Affluent: Challenges to Well-Being," *Current Directions in Psychological Science* 14, no. 1 (2005): 49–53.
4. Madeline Levine, *The Price of Privilege: How Parental Pressure and Material Advantage Are Creating a Generation of Disconnected and Unhappy Kids* (HarperCollins, 2006).
5. David Brooks, "The Moral Bucket List," *New York Times,* April 11, 2015, https://www.nytimes.com/2015/04/12/opinion/sunday/david-brooks-the-moral-bucket-list.html.

Chapter 1: The Adolescent Mental Health Crisis

1. Jonathan Haidt, *The Anxious Generation: How the Great Rewiring of Childhood Is Causing an Epidemic of Mental Illness* (New York: Penguin Press, 2024).
2. J. Ma et al., "Depression Treatment During Outpatient Visits by U.S. Children and Adolescents," *Journal of Adolescent Health* 37, no. 6 (2005): 434–42, https://doi.org/10.1016/j.jadohealth.2005.07.012.

3. It is possible that the increase was not due solely to rises in depression rates during that period. Raised awareness and/or reduced stigma could also contribute.
4. J. M. Twenge et al., "Birth Cohort Increases in Psychopathology Among Young Americans, 1938–2007: A Cross-temporal Meta-analysis of the MMPI," *Clinical Psychology Reviews* 30, no. 2 (2010): 145–54.
5. J. M. Twenge, "Time Period and Birth Cohort Differences in Depressive Symptoms in the U.S., 1982–2013," *Social Indicators Research* 121, no. 2 (2015): 437–54, https://doi.org/10.1007/s11205-014-0647-1.
6. C. L. Odgers, "The Great Rewiring: Is Social Media Really Behind an Epidemic of Teenage Mental Illness?," *Nature* 628, no. 8006 (March 29, 2024): 29–30, https//doi.org/10.1038/d41586-024-00902-2.
7. Kim, Brian, Mark Freeman, Trent Kajikawa, Honeiah Karimi, and Preston Magouirk. "First-year applications per applicant: Patterns of high-volume application activity at Common App." *Research brief, Common App* (2022), https://www.commonapp.org/about/reports-and-insights/first-year-applications-applicant.
8. AP Exam Volume Changes, 2013 and 2024 reports, https://reports.collegeboard.org/ap-program-results/data-archive.
9. National Center for Education Statistics. *Integrated Postsecondary Education Data System (IPEDS), Admissions Component, 2004–2023.* U.S. Department of Education. https://nces.ed.gov/ipeds/
10. Harvard University. *Common Data Set,* 2004–2023. Office of Institutional Research National Center for Education Statistics. *Integrated Postsecondary Education Data System (IPEDS), Admissions Component, 2005–2023.* U.S. Department of Education. Accessed February 26, 2026. https://nces.ed.gov/ipeds/
11. Rather than using the admissions rate for this graph, I chose to use the applicant-to-admitted-student ratio so that the parallels with depression can be easily seen (as the admission rate declines, the applicant-to-admitted-student ratio rises).
12. David Brooks, "We Are the Most Rejected Generation," *New York Times,* May 15, 2025, https://www.nytimes.com/2025/05/15/opinion/rejection-college-youth.html.
13. S. Paruthi et al., "Recommended Amount of Sleep for Pediatric Populations: A Consensus Statement of the American Academy of Sleep Medicine," *Journal of Clinical Sleep Medicine* 12, no. 6 (2016): 785–86.
14. S. S. Luthar and K. D'Avanzo, "Contextual Factors in Substance Use: A Study of Suburban and Inner-City Adolescents," *Development and Psychopathology* 11, no. 4 (1999): 845–67, https://doi.org/10.1017/S0954579499002357.
15. Thomas Steare et al., "The Association Between Academic Pressure and Adolescent Mental Health Problems: A Systematic Review," *Journal of Affective Disorders* 339 (October 2023): 302–17, https://doi.org/10.1016/j.jad.2023.07.028.
16. C. Rodway et al., "Children and Young People Who Die by Suicide: Childhood-Related Antecedents, Gender Differences and Service Contact," *BJPsych Open* 6, no. 3 (2020): e49o, https://doi.org/10.1192/bjo.2020.33.
17. D. C. Pope, *Doing School: How We Are Creating a Generation of Stressed-Out, Materialistic, and Miseducated Students* (Yale University Press, 2001).

18. Madeline Levine, *The Price of Privilege: How Parental Pressure and Material Advantage Are Creating a Generation of Disconnected and Unhappy Kids* (HarperCollins, 2006).
19. Challenge Success, *2024 Student Voice Report: Listening to and Learning from Students to Create More Equitable Schools* (Stanford University, 2024), https://challengesuccess.org/resources/2024-student-voice-report/.
20. P. Ishizuka, "Social Class, Gender, and Contemporary Parenting Standards in the United States: Evidence from a National Survey Experiment," *Social Forces* 98, no. 1 (2019): 31–58, https://doi.org/10.1093/sf/soy107.
21. B. Hansen et al., "In-Person Schooling and Youth Suicide: Evidence from School Calendars and Pandemic School Closures," National Bureau of Economic Research Report No. w30795, December 2022, https://www.nber.org/papers/w30795.
22. S. To et al., "Seasonal Variation in Suicide: Age Group and Summer Effects in the United States (2015–2020)," *BMC Psychiatry* 24, no. 856 (2024), https://doi.org/10.1186/s12888-024-06309-7.
23. L. Radhakrishnan, "Seasonal Trends in Emergency Department Visits for Mental and Behavioral Health Conditions Among Children and Adolescents Aged 5–17 Years—United States, January 2018—June 2023," *Morbidity and Mortality Weekly Report* 72, no. 38 (2023): 1032–40.
24. A. Nixon et al., "Psychiatric Admissions of Children and Adolescents Across School Periods and Daylight-Saving Transitions," *Journal of the Canadian Academy of Child and Adolescent Psychiatry* 30, no. 4 (November 2021): 226–35.
25. Y. Nishina et al., "Characteristics of Preteen Suicide in Japan," *JAMA Network Open* 8, no. 1 (2025): e2455471, https://doi.org/10.1001/jamanetworkopen.2024.55471.
26. R. Glenn Weaver et al., "The Impact of Summer Vacation on Children's Obesogenic Behaviors and Body Mass Index: A Natural Experiment," *International Journal of Behavioral Nutrition and Physical Activity* 17, no. 1 (2020): 153; Keith Brazendale et al., "Understanding Differences Between Summer vs. School Obesogenic Behaviors of Children: The Structured Days Hypothesis," *International Journal of Behavioral Nutrition and Physical Activity* 14, no. 1 (2017): 100.

Chapter 2: Depression in the Age of Pressure

1. L. S. Radloff, "The CES-D Scale: A Self-Report Depression Scale for Research in the General Population," *Applied Psychological Measurement* 1, no. 3 (1977): 385–401, https://doi.org/10.1177/014662167700100306.
2. For readability's sake, I will use the term *depression rate* for the remainder of the book rather than repeatedly writing "percentage who screened positive for moderate to severe symptoms of depression."
3. L. S. Rotenstein et al., "Prevalence of Depression, Depressive Symptoms, and Suicidal Ideation Among Medical Students: A Systematic Review and Meta-analysis," *JAMA* 316, no. 21 (December 6, 2016): 2214–36.

4. D. A. Mata et al., "Prevalence of Depression and Depressive Symptoms Among Resident Physicians: A Systematic Review and Meta-analysis," *JAMA* 314, no. 22 (December 8, 2015): 2373–83.
5. American Psychiatric Association, *Diagnostic and Statistical Manual of Mental Disorders: DSM-5,* 5th ed. (American Psychiatric Publishing, 2013).
6. Centers for Disease Control and Prevention, *2023 Youth Risk Behavior Survey Results* (U.S. Department of Health and Human Services, 2024), https//www.cdcgov/yrbs/results/2023-yrbs-results.html.
7. An important point—this was not true for headaches. While the vast majority of headache cases I saw were psychosocial in origin, some were caused by physical ailments such as migraine and in one case a brain tumor.
8. M. S. Askari et al., "Structure and Trends of Externalizing and Internalizing Psychiatric Symptoms and Gender Differences Among Adolescents in the US from 1991 to 2018," *Social Psychiatry and Psychiatric Epidemiology* 57, no. 4 (April 2022): 737–48, https://doi.org/10.1007/s00127-021-02189-4; erratum in *Social Psychiatry and Psychiatric Epidemiology* 58, no. 6 (2023): 987, https://doi.org/10.1007/s00127-023-02467-3.
9. D. Johnson et al., "Adult Mental Health Outcomes of Adolescent Depression: A Systematic Review," *Depression and Anxiety* 35, no. 8 (August 2018): 700–716.
10. S. K. Lipson et al., "Increased Rates of Mental Health Service Utilization by U.S. College Students: 10-Year Population-Level Trends (2007–2017)," *Psychiatric Services* 70, no. 1 (January 1, 2019): 60–63, https://doi.org/10.1176/appi.ps.201800332.
11. E. A. Pfau et al., "College Student Mental Health: Exploring Depression, Anxiety, and Mindsets in First-Year STEM Students," *Journal of Chemical Education* 101, no. 12 (2024): 5288–96, https://doi.org/10.1021/acs.jchemed.4c00791.
12. B. T. Williams et al., "Efficacy and Acceptability of Third-Wave Psychotherapies in the Treatment of Depression: A Systematic Review and Meta-analysis," *Frontiers in Psychiatry* 14 (2023):1189970, https://doi.org/10.3389/fpsyt.2023.1189970.
13. National Institute for Health and Care Research (NIHR), "Combined Drug and Psychological Therapies May Be Most Effective for Depression," *NIHR Evidence,* March 7, 2020, https://evidence.nihr.ac.uk/alert/combined-drug-and-psychological-therapies-may-be-most-effective-for-depression.
14. These parental beliefs are not in any way unique to this population and occur across many cultures. I am simply relating my own personal experience with medical students.
15. I need to credit Surgeon General Murthy here. While I believe his diagnosis of social media as the primary cause of the mental health crisis is incorrect, I do appreciate his focus on prevention of mental illness.
16. R. A. Zuckerbrot et al., "Guidelines for Adolescent Depression in Primary Care (GLAD-PC): I. Identification, Assessment, and Initial Management," *Pediatrics* 120, no. 5 (November 1, 2007): e1299–312; A. H. Cheung et al., "Guidelines for Adolescent Depression in Primary Care (GLAD-PC): II. Treatment and Ongoing Management," *Pediatrics* 120, no. 5 (November 1, 2007): e1313–26.

17. D. Storey, "Suicide Plagues Student-Athletes," *Psychiatrist.com,* April 18, 2024, https://www.psychiatrist.com/news/suicide-plagues-student-athletes/.

Chapter 3: Understanding Anxiety

1. J. M. Twenge et al., "Birth Cohort Increases in Psychopathology Among Young Americans, 1938–2007: A Cross-temporal Meta-analysis of the MMPI," *Clinical Psychology Review* 30, no. 2 (2010): 145–54, https://doi.org/10.1016/j.cpr.2009.10.005.
2. O. Sappenfield et al., *Adolescent Mental and Behavioral Health, 2023,* NSCH Data Brief, October 2024, https://www.ncbi.nlm.nih.gov/books/NBK608531.
3. K. R. Merikangas et al., "Lifetime Prevalence of Mental Disorders in U.S. Adolescents: Results from the National Comorbidity Survey Replication—Adolescent Supplement (NCS-A)," *Journal of the American Academy of Child and Adolescent Psychiatry* 49, no. 10 (October 2010): 980–89.
4. American College Health Association, "American College Health Association–National College Health Assessment, Spring 2008 Reference Group Data Report (Abridged)," *Journal of American College Health* 57, no. 5 (2008): 477–88; *American College Health Association, American College Health Association-National College Health Assessment II: Reference Group Executive Summary Spring 2019* (American College Health Association, 2019); American College Health Association, *American College Health Association-National College Health Assessment III: Reference Group Executive Summary Fall 2022* (American College Health Association, 2023).
5. Using a screening tool called the Spielberger State-Trait Anxiety Inventory. (I later changed to utilize another widely used and shorter survey, the Generalized Anxiety Disorder-7 [GAD-7] scale.) As with the depression scales I described in the last chapter, you can't make a diagnosis of anxiety with this instrument, but you can identify the level of symptoms that people are experiencing. Anything from moderate to above is viewed as being likely to be associated with a diagnosis of an anxiety disorder.
6. T. Steare et al., "The Association Between Academic Pressure and Adolescent Mental Health Problems: A Systematic Review," *Journal of Affective Disorders* 339 (2023): 302–17, https://doi.org/10.1016/j.jad.2023.07.028.
7. L. Cardona et al., "Contributing Factors to the Rise in Adolescent Anxiety and Associated Mental Health Disorders: A Narrative Review of Current Literature," *Journal of Child and Adolescent Psychiatric Nursing* 37, no. 1 (2024): 3–12, https://doi.org/10.1111/jcap.12345.
8. M. B. Geisz and M. Nakashian, *Adolescent Wellness: Current Perspectives and Future Opportunities in Research, Policy, and Practice* (Robert Wood Johnson Foundation, 2018).
9. H. A. Franke, "Toxic Stress: Effects, Prevention and Treatment," *Children (Basel)* 1, no. 3 (2014): 390–402, https://doi.org/10.3390/children1030390; "Toxic Stress," Center on the Developing Child at Harvard University, 2023, https://developingchild.harvard.edu/key-concept/toxic-stress/; M. Bucci et al., "Toxic

Stress in Children and Adolescents," *Advances in Pediatrics* 63, no. 1 (August 1, 2016): 403–28.

10. Charles D. Spielberger, *State-Trait Anxiety Inventory for Adults* (Palo Alto, CA: Consulting Psychologists Press, 1983).
11. This can be introduced earlier in this sequence, but my inclination is to not rush to use it as I think it's more likely to be rejected if some kind of plan hasn't emerged.
12. Another popular breathing technique is box or square breathing, 4-4-4-4. It is used by the Navy SEALs. Breathe in to four, hold for four, exhale to four, hold for four, repeat.
13. A. C. James et al., "Cognitive Behavioral Therapy for Anxiety Disorders in Children and Adolescents," *Cochrane Database of Systematic Reviews,* no. 11 (2020): art. no. CD013162.
14. Despite its widespread acceptance, it's important to note that CBT has received a range of criticisms, including that it is culturally biased toward Western individualistic cultures, overemphasizes cognition, and is simplistic and reductionistic, focusing too much on thoughts and not on areas such as meaning and values.
15. S. Fang and D. Ding, "A Meta-analysis of the Efficacy of Acceptance and Commitment Therapy for Children," *Journal of Contextual Behavioral Science* 15 (January 1, 2020): 225–34; M. P. Twohig and M. E. Levin, "Acceptance and Commitment Therapy as a Treatment for Anxiety and Depression: A Review," *Psychiatric Clinics of North America* 40, no. 4 (2017): 751–70, https://doi.org/10.1016/j.psc.2017.08.009; J. G. L. A-Tjak et al., "A Meta-analysis of the Efficacy of Acceptance and Commitment Therapy for Clinically Relevant Mental and Physical Health Problems," *Psychotherapy and Psychosomatics* 84, no. 1 (2015): 30–36, https://doi.org/10.1159/000365764.
16. M. M. Linehan et al., "Cognitive-Behavioral Treatment of Chronically Parasuicidal Borderline Patients," *Archives of General Psychiatry* 48, no. 12 (1991): 1060–64, https://doi.org/10.1001/archpsyc.1991.01810360024003.
17. While anxiety is not as strongly associated with suicidality as depression is, in teens with clinical anxiety suicidality remains common.
18. The recommended approaches are consistent with guidelines from Psychological First Aid, an evidence-based approach for providing psychosocial support in the aftermath of disasters, crises, and traumatic events. This approach was developed by the National Child Traumatic Stress Network and the National Center for PTSD. It has been endorsed by the World Health Organization, the United Nations, and the International Red Cross among others. It promotes focusing initially on calming and emotional support rather than jumping too quickly to problem-solving. Guide, Field Operations. "Psychological First Aid." (2006).

Chapter 4: My Initiative to Combat Depression, Anxiety, and Toxic Stress in My Students

1. L. N. Dyrbye et al., "Burnout and Suicidal Ideation Among U.S. Medical Students," *Annals of Internal Medicine* 149, no. 5 (2008): 334–41; L. N. Dyrbye

et al., "Systematic Review of Depression, Anxiety, and Other Indicators of Psychological Distress Among U.S. and Canadian Medical Students," *Academic Medicine* 81, no. 4 (2006): 354–73.

2. L. S. Robins et al., "The Effect of Pass/Fail Grading and Weekly Quizzes on First-Year Students' Performances and Satisfaction," *Academic Medicine* 70 (1995): 327–29; D. E. Rohe et al., "The Benefits of Pass-Fail Grading on Stress, Mood, and Group Cohesion in Medical Students," *Mayo Clinic Proceedings* 81 (2006): 1443–48; R. A. Bloodgood et al., "A Change to Pass/Fail Grading in the First Two Years at One Medical School Results in Improved Psychological Well-Being," *Academic Medicine* 84 (2009): 655–62.
3. Viktor E. Frankl, *Man's Search for Meaning* (Beacon Press, 1959).
4. "SLU Medical Students Form Incubator to Foster Biomedical Innovation," Saint Louis University, June 15, 2016, https://www.slu.edu/news/2016/june/medlaunch.php.
5. "To Build a 'More Humane' Medical School, Saint Louis University Looks to Its Students," St. Louis Public Radio, August 4, 2016, https://www.stlpr.org/health-science-environment/2016-08-04/to-build-a-more-humane-medical-school-saint-louis-university-looks-to-its-students.
6. S. Slavin, "Reflections on a decade leading a medical student well-being initiative." *Academic Medicine* 94, no. 6 (2019): 771–774.
7. Association of American Medical Colleges, "Year Two Questionnaire (Y2Q)," 2025, https://www.aamc.org/data-reports/students-residents/report/year-two-questionnaire-y2q.
8. M. G. Calvo and A. Gutiérrez-García, "Cognition and Stress," in *Stress: Concepts, Cognition, Emotion, and Behavior*, ed. G. Fink (Academic Press, 2016), https://doi.org/10.1016/b978-0-12-800951-2.00016-9.
9. A. Kulshreshtha et al., "Association of Stress with Cognitive Function Among Older Black and White US Adults," *JAMA Network Open* 6, no. 3 (2023): e231860, https://doi.org/10.1001/jamanetworkopen.2023.1860.

Chapter 5: Problematic Mindsets

1. T. Curran and A. P. Hill, "Perfectionism Is Increasing over Time: A Meta-analysis of Birth Cohort Differences from 1989 to 2016," *Psychological Bulletin* 145, no. 4 (April 2019): 410.
2. R. B. Slaney et al., "Perfectionism: Its Measurement and Career Relevance," *Journal of Career Assessment* 3, no. 3 (1995): 279–97.
3. K. G. Rice et al., "The Short Form of the Revised Almost Perfect Scale," *Journal of Personality Assessment* 96, no. 3 (2014: 368–79, https://doi.org/10.1080/00223891.2013.838172.
4. E. Pfau et al., "College Student Mental Health: Exploring Depression, Anxiety, and Mindsets in First-Year STEM Students," *Journal of Chemical Education* 101, no. 12 (2024): 5288–5296.
5. D. Lester and T. Moderski, "The Impostor Phenomenon in Adolescents," *Psychological Reports* 76, no. 2 (1995): art. no. 466; R. Garba et al., "The

Impostor Phenomenon and Mental Health," in *The Impostor Phenomenon: Psychological Research, Theory, and Interventions,* ed. K. Cokley (American Psychological Association, 2024), https://doi.org/10.1037/0000397-004.

6. P. R. Clance and S. A. Imes, "The Impostor Phenomenon in High Achieving Women: Dynamics and Therapeutic Intervention," *Psychotherapy: Theory, Research and Practice* 15, no. 3 (1978): 241–47.
7. P. R. Clance, *The Impostor Phenomenon: When Success Makes You Feel Like a Fake* (Toronto: Bantam Books, 1985).
8. M. R. Leary et al., "The Impostor Phenomenon: Self-Perceptions, Reflected Appraisals, and Interpersonal Strategies," *Journal of Personality* 68, no. 4 (2000): 725–56, https://doi.org/10.1111/1467-6494.00114.
9. M. Dahlin et al., "Performance-Based Self-Esteem and Burnout in a Cross-sectional Study of Medical Students," *Medical Teacher* 29, no. 1 (2007): 43–48, https://doi.org/10.1080/01421590601175309.
10. K. S. Hu et al., "Maladaptive Perfectionism, Impostorism, and Cognitive Distortions: Threats to the Mental Health of Pre-clinical Medical Students," *Academic Psychiatry* 43, no. 4 (August 15, 2019): 381–85.

Chapter 6: Cognitive Distortions

1. A. T. Beck, "Thinking and Depression: I. Idiosyncratic Content and Cognitive Distortions," *Archives of General Psychiatry* 9, no. 4 (1963): 324–33.
2. A. T. Beck et al., *Cognitive Therapy of Depression* (Guilford Press, 1979).
3. Epictetus, *The Handbook (The Enchiridion),* trans. N. White (Hackett, 1983).
4. M. Aurelius, *The Meditations of Marcus Aurelius.* trans. G. Long (Dover Publications, 1997).
5. Nhat Hánh and Melvin McLeod, *Your True Home: The Everyday Wisdom of Thich Nhat Hanh* (Shambhala, 2011).
6. K. C. Bathina et al., "Individuals with Depression Express More Distorted Thinking on Social Media," *Nature Human Behaviour* 5 (2021): 458–66, https://doi.org/10.1038/s41562-021-01050-7.
7. A. Ray, *Mindfulness: Living in the Moment, Living in the Breath* (Inner Light, 2015).
8. When speaking in front of medical audiences, I often ask people to raise their hands if they have a meditation practice of fifteen minutes or more a day. In no audience have I ever seen more than 3 percent raise their hands, even in California.

Chapter 7: Goal Disruption Theory

1. J. Siegel, "What Is a Goal Disruption?," in "Goal Disruption Theory: A Theoretical Startup," 2013, http://www.gdtheory.com/what-is-a-goal-disruption.html.
2. W. C. Ameden et al., "The Role of Planfulness for Well-Being, Stress, and Goal

Disruption During COVID-19," *Frontiers in Psychology* 15 (February 8, 2024): 1224451.

Chapter 8: Your Kid in School

1. John Dewey, "My Pedagogic Creed," *School Journal* 54, no. 3 (January 16, 1897): 77–80. Also available in the Informal Education Archives, https://infed.org/mobi/john-dewey-my-pedagogical-creed/; John Dewey, *The School and Society: Being Three Lectures* (University of Chicago Press, 1899); John Dewey, *The Child and the Curriculum* (University of Chicago Press, 1902).
2. John Dewey, *Democracy and Education: An Introduction to the Philosophy of Education* (Macmillan, 1916).
3. Council of the Great City Schools, *Student Testing in America's Great City Schools: An Inventory and Preliminary Analysis* (Council of the Great City Schools, October 2015), https://files.eric.ed.gov/fulltext/ED569198.pdf.
4. N. K. Segool et al., "Heightened Test Anxiety Among Young Children: Elementary School Students' Anxious Responses to High-Stakes Testing," *Psychology in the Schools* 50, no. 5 (May 2013): 489–99.
5. B. D. Jones and R. J. Egley, "Voices from the Frontlines: Teachers' Perceptions of High-Stakes Testing," *Education Policy Analysis Archives* 12 (2004): 39, https://doi.org/10.14507/epaa.v12n39.2004.
6. D. Berliner, "Rational Responses to High Stakes Testing: The Case of Curriculum Narrowing and the Harm That Follows," *Cambridge Journal of Education* 41, no. 3 (2011): 287–302, https://doi.org/10.1080/0305764X.2011.607151.
7. E. L. Deci et al., "Motivation and Education: The Self-Determination Perspective," *Educational Psychology* 26, nos. 3–4 (1991): 325–46; H. Jang et al., "Engaging Students in Learning Activities: It Is Not Autonomy Support or Structure but Autonomy Support and Structure," *Journal of Educational Psychology* 102, no. 3 (2010): 588–600; C. P. Niemiec and R. M. Ryan, "Autonomy, Competence, and Relatedness in the Classroom: Applying Self-Determination Theory to Educational Practice," *Theory and Research in Education* 7, no. 2 (2009): 133–44; M. Vansteenkiste et al., "Motivating Learning, Performance, and Persistence: The Synergistic Effects of Intrinsic Goal Contents and Autonomy-Supportive Contexts," *Journal of Personality and Social Psychology* 87, no. 2 (2004): 246–60.
8. J. L. Howard et al., "Student Motivation and Associated Outcomes: A Meta-analysis from Self-Determination Theory," *Perspectives on Psychological Science* 16, no. 6 (November 2021): 1300–1323.
9. H. Cooper, *Homework* (Longman, 1989); H. Cooper et al., "Does Homework Improve Academic Achievement? A Synthesis of Research, 1987–2003," *Review of Educational Research* 76, no. 1 (2006): 1–62, https://doi.org/10.3102/00346543076001001.
10. T. Walker, "If Elementary Schools Say No to Homework, What Takes Its Place? No Homework Policies Are Popular, but Educators Are Working with Parents

on Stress-Free Ways to Keep Learning Going," *NEA Today,* January 26, 2017, https://www.nea.org/nea-today/all-news-articles/if-elementary-schools-say-no-homework-what-takes-its-place.

11. M. Galloway et al., "Nonacademic Effects of Homework in Privileged, High-Performing High Schools," *Journal of Experimental Education* 81, no. 4 (2013): 490–510, https://doi.org/10.1080/00220973.2012.745469.
12. Steven Yoder, "Kids Are Failing Algebra. The Solution? Slow Down," *Hechinger Report,* July 13, 2021, https://hechingerreport.org/kids-are-failing-algebra-the-solution-slow-down/.
13. U.S. Department of Education, National Center for Education Statistics, "Status Dropout Rates," in *The Condition of Education* (NCES, 2022), https://nces.ed.gov/programs/coe/indicator/coj.
14. U.S. Department of Education, Office for Civil Rights, *2020–21 Civil Rights Data Collection: Student Discipline and School Climate* (U.S. Department of Education, November 2023), https://nces.ed.gov/programs/raceindicators/indicator_rda.asp.
15. M. Hanson, "College Enrollment and Student Demographic Statistics," Education Data Initiative, July 26, 2022, https://educationdata.org/college-enrollment-statistics.
16. M. M. Schwartze et al., "Excessive Boredom Among Adolescents: A Comparison Between Low and High Achievers," *PLoS ONE* 15, no. 11 (2020): e0241671, https://doi.org/10.1371/journal.pone.0241671.
17. E. H. Weybright et al., "More Bored Today Than Yesterday? National Trends in Adolescent Boredom from 2008 to 2017," *Journal of Adolescent Health* 66, no. 3 (March 2020): 360–65, https://doi.org/10.1016/j.jadohealth.2019.09.021.
18. A. Chin et al., "Bored in the USA: Experience Sampling and Boredom in Everyday Life," *Emotion* 17, no. 2 (2017): 359–68, https://doi.org/10.1037/emo0000232; D. M. Ndetei et al., "Boredom—Understanding the Emotion and Its Impact on Our Lives: An African Perspective," *Frontiers in Sociology* 8 (June 29, 2023): 1213190, https://doi.org/10.3389/fsoc.2023.1213190.
19. S. S. Luthar and B. E. Becker, "Privileged but Pressured? A Study of Affluent Youth," *Child Development* 73, no. 5 (2002): 1593–610, https://doi.org/10.1111/1467-8624.00492; S. S. Luthar and S. J. Latendresse, "Children of the Affluent: Challenges to Well-Being," *Current Directions in Psychological Science* 14, no. 1 (2005):49–53, https://doi.org/10.1111/j.0963-7214.2005.00333.x.
20. Frank Bruni, *Where You Go Is Not Who You'll Be: An Antidote to the College Admissions Mania* (Grand Central Publishing, 2015); William Deresiewicz, *Excellent Sheep: The Miseducation of the American Elite and the Way to a Meaningful Life* (Free Press, 2014).
21. Malcolm Gladwell, *David and Goliath: Underdogs, Misfits, and the Art of Battling Giants* (Little, Brown, 2013).
22. Harvard University, Graduate School of Education, "School-Family College Admissions Compact," last reviewed August 2019, https://mcc.gse.harvard.edu/resources-for-educators/school-family-compact.

23. Suniya Luthar, "The Mental Price of Affluence," interview, transcript of episode 18 of *Speaking of Psychology* podcast, 2014, https://www.apa.org/news/podcasts/speaking-of-psychology/affluence.

Chapter 9: Your Kid After School

1. NFHS, "Participation in High School Sports Tops Eight Million for First Time in 2023–24," press release, September 10, 2024, NFHS website, https://nfhs.org/stories/participation-in-high-school-sports-tops-eight-million-for-first-time-in-2023-24.
2. J. Solomon, "Project Play Survey: Family Spending on Youth Sports Rises 46% over Five Years," Aspen Institute, March 3, 2025, https://projectplay.org/news/2025/2/24/project-play-survey-family-spending-on-youth-sports-rises-46-over-five-years.
3. B. J. Erickson et al., "Trends in Medial Ulnar Collateral Ligament Reconstruction in the United States: A Retrospective Review of a Large Private-Payer Database from 2007 to 2011," *American Journal of Sports Medicine* 43 (2015): 1770–74.
4. H. Korbey, "The Revolution: More Families Are Seeking One-on-One Help for Their Kids. What Does That Tell Us About 21st-Century Education?," *Education Next* 25, no. 1 (2025): 16–21, https://www.educationnext.org/the-tutoring-revolution-more-families-seek-one-on-one-help-education; Global Private Tutoring Market to Reach $201.8 Billion by 2026. https://finance.yahoo.com/news/global-private-tutoring-market-reach-145300655.html.
5. J. S. Brenner and Council on Sports Medicine and Fitness, "Overuse Injuries, Overtraining, and Burnout in Child and Adolescent Athletes," *Pediatrics* 119, no. 6 (June 1, 2007): 1242–45; H. L. Glandorf et al., "Mental and Physical Health Outcomes of Burnout in Athletes: A Systematic Review and Meta-analysis," *International Review of Sport and Exercise Psychology* 18, no. 1 (January 2, 2025): 372–416; R. Mancine et al., "Disordered Eating and Eating Disorders in Adolescent Athletes," *Spartan Medical Research Journal* 4, no. 2 (January 30, 2020): 11595.
6. M. Hirshkowitz et al., "National Sleep Foundation's Sleep Time Duration Recommendations: Methodology and Results Summary," *Sleep Health* 1, no. 1 (March 1, 2015): 40–43.
7. D. Dawson and K. Reid, "Fatigue, Alcohol and Performance Impairment," *Nature* 388, no. 235 (1997), https://doi.org/10.1038/40775.
8. D. W. Beebe et al., "Attention, Learning, and Arousal of Experimentally Sleep-Restricted Adolescents in a Simulated Classroom," *Journal of Adolescent Health* 47, no. 5 (November 1, 2010): 523–25.
9. G. Medic et al., "Short-and Long-Term Health Consequences of Sleep Disruption," *Nature and Science of Sleep,* May 19, 2017, 151–61.
10. S. S. Luthar et al., "'I Can, Therefore I Must': Fragility in the Upper-Middle Classes," *Developmental Psychopathology* 25, no. 4, pt. 2 (2013): 1529–49, https://doi.org/10.1017/S0954579413000758.

11. T. D. Shanafelt et al., "Changes in Burnout and Satisfaction with Work-Life Balance in Physicians and the General US Working Population Between 2011 and 2014," *Mayo Clinic Proceedings* 90, no. 12 (December 1, 2015): 1600–1613; A. Getie et al., "Global Prevalence and Contributing Factors of Nurse Burnout: An Umbrella Review of Systematic Review and Meta-analysis," *BMC Nursing* 24, no. 1 (May 26, 2025): 596.
12. C. Maslach and S. Jackson. "The measurement of experienced burnout." *Journal of Organizational Behavior* 2, no. 2 (1981): 99–113.
13. Office of the Surgeon General, *Parents Under Pressure: The U.S. Surgeon General's Advisory on the Mental Health and Well-Being of Parents* (U.S. Department of Health and Human Services, 2024), https://www.hhs.gov/sites/default/files/parents-under-pressure.pdf.
14. Patrick Ishizuka, "Social Class, Gender, and Contemporary Parenting Standards in the United States: Evidence from a National Survey Experiment," *Social Forces* 98, no. 1 (September 2019): 31–58, https://doi.org/10.1093/sf/soy107.
15. S. B. Wolicki et al., "Mental Health of Parents and Primary Caregivers by Sex and Associated Child Health Indicators," *Adversity and Resilience Science* 2, no. 2 (June 2021): 125–39.
16. S. Y. Rueger et al., "Relationship Between Multiple Sources of Perceived Social Support and Psychological and Academic Adjustment in Early Adolescence: Comparisons Across Gender," *Journal of Youth and Adolescence* 39, no. 1 (2010): 47–61, https://doi.org/10.1007/s10964-008-9368-6; P. E. Jose et al., "Does Social Connectedness Promote a Greater Sense of Well-Being in Adolescence over Time?," *Journal of Research on Adolescence* 22, no. 2 (June 2012): 235–51; S. S. Luthar and B. E. Becker, "Privileged but Pressured? A Study of Affluent Youth," *Child Development* 73, no. 5 (2002): 1593–610.
17. "The Power of Play with Dr. Peter Gray," *The Child Psych Podcast,* episode #105, November 6, 2024.
18. T. Shlain, *24/6: Giving Up Screens One Day a Week to Get More Time, Creativity, and Connection* (Gallery Books, 2019).

Chapter 10: Giving Kids More Control, More Choice, and Opportunities to Find Connection, Meaning, and Joy

1. E. L. Deci and R. M. Ryan, "The 'What' and 'Why' of Goal Pursuits: Human Needs and the Self-Determination of Behavior," *Psychological Inquiry* 11, no. 4 (2000): 227–268.
2. R. M. Ryan and E. L. Deci, "Self-Determination Theory and the Facilitation of Intrinsic Motivation, Social Development, and Well-Being," *American Psychologist* 55, no. 1 (2000): 68–78; J. L. Howard et al., "Student Motivation and Associated Outcomes: A Meta-analysis from Self-Determination Theory," *Perspectives on Psychological Science* 16, no. 6 (November 2021): 1300–1323; Z. Liu et al., "Basic Psychological Need Satisfaction and Depression in Adolescents During the COVID-19 Pandemic: The Mediating Roles of Feelings of Safety and Rumination," *Child Psychiatry and Human Development* 55, no. 1

(February 2024): 219–26; J. L. Howard et al., "Student Motivation and Associated Outcomes: A Meta-analysis from Self-Determination Theory," *Perspectives on Psychological Science* 16, no. 6 (November 2021): 1300–1323; Z. Liu et al., "Basic Psychological Need Satisfaction and Depression in Adolescents During the COVID-19 Pandemic: The Mediating Roles of Feelings of Safety and Rumination," *Child Psychiatry and Human Development* 55, no. 1 (February 2024): 219–26.

3. Stuart J. Slavin and John T. Chibnall, "Finding the Why, Changing the How: Improving the Mental Health of Medical Students, Residents, and Physicians," *Academic Medicine* 91, no. 9 (2016): 1194–1196.
4. J. M. Twenge, "The Evidence for Generation Me and Against Generation We," *Emerging Adulthood* 1, no. 1 (March 2013): 11–16.

Supplemental Resources

1. S. Jordan, "SLU Med Students Protest Dismissal of Dean, Dr. Stuart Slavin Takes Fall for Negative Accreditation Report," *St. Louis American,* May 15, 2017, https://www.stlamerican.com/news/local_news/slu-med-students-protest-dismissal-of-dean-dr-stuart-slavin-takes-fall-for-negative-accreditation/article_76cf014a-f52d-11e8-82d2-e3ed4c5d6234.html; St. Louis Public Radio, "SLU's Medical School Removes Dean Lauded for Preventing Student Depression," *NPR,* May 10, 2017, https://www.stlpr.org/health-science-environment/2017-05-10/slus-medical-school-removes-dean-lauded-for-preventing-student-depression.
2. Kurt Lewin, *Field Theory in Social Science: Selected Theoretical Papers,* ed. D. Cartwright (Harper and Row, 1951).
3. Personal communication with Mike Nicholson.
4. D. St. George, "Later School Start Times in Fairfax Could Set Trend as Experts Call for More Teen Sleep," *Washington Post,* October 24, 2014, https://www.washingtonpost.com/local/education/later-school-start-times-in-fairfax-could-set-trend-as-experts-call-for-more-teen-sleep/2014/10/24/421e7bc8-5ba1-11e4-b812-38518ae74c67_story.html.
5. C. Rowe, "Seattle Board Approves Later Start Times for Schools," *Seattle Times,* November 19, 2015, https://www.seattletimes.com/seattle-news/education/seattle-board-approves-later-start-times-for-schools/.
6. K. Wahlstrom, "Changing Times: Findings from the First Longitudinal Study of Later High School Start Times," *NASSP Bulletin* 86, no. 633 (December 2002): 3–21; Kyla Wahlstrom et al., "Examining the Impact of Later High School Start Times on the Health and Academic Performance of High School Students: A Multi-site Study," February 2014, University Digital Conservancy, https://hdl.handle.net/11299/162769.

Index

A

Abeles, Vicki, 13
academic performance
  change and, 258
  as identity, 115–18
  pressure and, 87–89
academic pressure. *See* pressure
acceptance and commitment therapy (ACT), 39, 64, 65
Accreditation Council for Graduate Medical Education, 254
adaptive perfectionism, 104, 105–6
Advanced Placement (AP) courses, 10, 174
Alagic, Asmira, 37
allies, enlisting, 256–57
all-or-nothing thinking, 127
Almost Perfect Scale, 101
American Academy of Child and Adolescent Psychiatry, 52, 64
American Academy of Pediatrics, 52
American College Health Association, 50
American Psychiatric Association (APA), 30, 43
American Psychological Association, 64
analyzing the evidence technique, 139–41, 145–46, 147–48
antidepressants, 39
anxiety
  causes of, 19–20, 51, 68, 261
  clinical, 57–58, 63–67
  cognitive distortions and, 126
  dependency, 67
  effects of, 56, 58
  example of, 46–49
  extracurricular activities and, 205
  normal, 53, 54, 60–63
  parental support for, 60–67
  in parents, 62–63
  prevalence of, xv, 5, 50–53, 72
  professional evaluation for, 63–64
  SLU initiative to combat, 71–91
  symptoms of, 54, 57–58, 60–61, 63
  as systemic problem, 68
  treatment for, 52, 64–66

Aspen Institute, 198
Association of American Medical Colleges (AAMC), 86
autonomy, 83, 172–73, 222, 225–27, 229–35
awareness, raising, 258–59

B

Beck, Aaron, 64, 125, 126
behaviors, externalizing vs. internalizing, 35–36
biological stress response, 53, 55–57
black-and-white thinking. *See* all-or-nothing thinking
block scheduling, 178, 180, 263–64
borderline personality disorder (BPD), 65
boys, as special risk group, 178
breathing techniques, 62
Brooks, David, xvi, 12
Bruni, Frank, 185
Buddhism, 125
bullying, 15
burnout, 206–8, 215–18
Burns, David D., 126
Bush, George W., 169

C

Catalyst Learning Labs, 181
catastrophizing, 123, 124, 129–30, 142, 147, 156, 157
causation vs. correlation, 7–8
Centers for Disease Control (CDC), 22, 31
Challenge Success, 21
change
  advocating for, 251–54
  areas for, 262–67
  bringing about, 255–62
  costs and, 259
  effort required for, 81
  need for, 251
  obstacles to, 79–81, 253–54, 261–62
  parents' role in, 251–52
  possibility of, 253, 260, 267
Chibnall, John, 27–28, 71–72, 83–84, 223
Chicago, University of, 167
choice
  giving more, 83, 91, 229–35
  lack of, xxi, 225–27
  See also self-determination theory
Cincinnati Children's Hospital, 266
Clance, Pauline, 112
Clance Impostor Phenomenon Scale (CIPS), 112
cognitive behavioral therapy (CBT), 38–39, 64–65, 125, 133
cognitive defusion, 65
cognitive distortions
  all-or-nothing thinking, 127
  catastrophizing, 129–30
  categorizing, 126
  development of, xx
  disbelief, 130–31
  effects of, 125, 126–27, 131–32
  fortune-telling, 129
  magnification, 127
  mind reading, 130
  overgeneralization, 128
  personalization and self-blame, 128
  tunnel vision, 128–29
cognitive restructuring
  benefits of, 39, 77, 109, 148
  examples of, 141–48
  overview of, 132–35
  steps in, 135–41
collaboration, 82, 240
college
  anxiety and, 50
  depression and, 37
college applications
  average number of, 9–10
  to elite universities, 10–12
  parents and, 186–88, 232, 237
comparison, toxic, 119–21, 205, 227
competence, 222, 227–28, 235–39

control
giving more, 83, 91, 229–35
lack of, xxi
See also self-determination theory
Cooper, Harris, 175
correlation vs. causation, 7–8
COVID-19 pandemic, 10, 14, 15, 21, 164, 180–81
Crisis Text Line, 40
cyberbullying, 15

D

Deci, Edward, 222
Democracy and Education, 167
depersonalization, 206
depression
in adulthood, 36–37
causes of, 19–20, 30–31, 42–45, 261
cognitive distortions and, 126
diagnosing, 30
endogenous vs. reactive, 30–31
environment's role in, 30–32
extracurricular activities and, 205
increasing pressure and, 9–12
masking of, 28, 32
parental support and, 40–41
prevalence of, xv, 5–7, 27–29, 31, 72
preventing, 43–44
professional evaluation for, 38
recognizing, 32–36
research on, 27–29
shame and, 41–42
SLU initiative to combat, 71–91
suicide and, 39–40
symptoms accompanying, 7, 28, 30, 32–36
as systemic problem, 42–45
taking action, 36–37
treatment for, 38–39, 42
Deresiewicz, William, 185–86
Dewey, John, 167–68
Diagnostic and Statistical Manual of Mental Disorders (DSM), 30, 57
dialectical behavior therapy (DBT), 39, 64, 65–66
digital technology. *See* social media and digital technology
disbelief, 130–31
discrepancy technique, 139, 140, 145, 147
Dodson, John Dillingham, 88

E

eating disorders, 100, 205
educational theory, 167–68
electives
choosing, 231
increasing time for, 264
Environmental Protection Agency (EPA), 44
Epictetus, 125
eustress, 55–56
Every Student Succeeds Act, 169
extracurricular activities
benefits of, 203
choosing, 231
coordinating academic demands and, 265
effects of excessive, 203–10
parental support and, 210–15
time spent on, 16, 23–25, 195–201

F

family time
emphasizing importance of, 210–11, 241
lack of, 208–9
fear
of failure, 113
impostor phenomenon and, 113
Feeling Good: The New Mood Therapy, 126
feelings
goal expectation violations and, 153–54
labeling, 137–38, 144–45, 147

feelings (*cont'd*)
  maladaptive perfectionism and, 122
  noticing, 135–37, 144, 146
Fendell, Ginny, 132
field theory, 255
fight-or-flight mechanism, 53, 55–57
Flint, Michigan, 44–45
fortune-telling, 129
4-7-8 breathing, 62
Frankl, Viktor, 78
Freudenberger, Herbert, 206

G

generalized anxiety disorder (GAD), 57–58. *See also* anxiety
Gladwell, Malcolm, 186
goal expectation violations
  definition of, 150–51, 152
  effects of, 151–57
  example of, 149–50
  parental support and, 157–65
  personality traits and, 158
  preventing, 162–65
grades
  competition for, 74, 76–77
  focus on, 173–74
  identity and, 80–81
  implementing changes in, 267
  maladaptive perfectionism and, 17, 100
  pass/fail, 75, 76–77, 80–81
gratitude
  journal, 217
  practicing and expressing, 218
Gray, Peter, 209
Great Recession of 2007 to 2009, 8

H

Haidt, Jonathan, 3, 4–6, 8, 24
Hanna, Mona, 44–45
Harvard University, 10–12, 186
Healthy Minds Study, 37
High Tech High, 180
homework
  autonomy and, 230
  recommended amount of, 175
  reducing, 263
  time spent on, 16, 174–76
Hurley Medical Center, 45
hypervigilance, 155

I

Imes, Suzanne, 112
impostor phenomenon, 110–14, 122
isolation, 34

J

Jackson, Jay, 13
Johnson, Ned, 201–2, 230
joy
  finding, 91, 242–45
  importance of, 221–22
  lack of, xxi

L

lead, in drinking water, 44–45
learning
  differences, 177–78
  passive, 170–71, 179
  project-based, 180
  self-directed, 166, 168, 265–66
Learning InspirED, 166, 257
Leary Impostorism Scale (LIS), 112
Levine, Madeline, xvi, 20
Lewin, Kurt, 255
Linehan, Marsha M., 65
Louisiana Tech University, 198
love, unconditional, 120–21, 163, 184
Luthar, Suniya, xvi, 19–20, 51, 184, 188, 205, 213

M

magnification, 127
Mahoney, Jim, 251, 255

Making Caring Common Project, 186
maladaptive perfectionism
  definition of, 99
  effects of, 17
  emotions and, 122
  managing, 109–10
  measuring, 101–4
  prevalence of, 17, 98
  preventing, 108–9
  recognizing, 100–101, 106–8
  self-oriented, 99–101, 104
Man's Search for Meaning, 78
Marcus Aurelius, 125
Maslach, Christina, 206
Mayo Medical School, 77
meaning
  finding, 78, 82–83, 91, 242–45
  importance of, 221–22
  lack of, xxi
medications
  antianxiety, 66
  antidepressant, 39
MEDLaunch, 82
mental health crisis
  causes of, 3, 7–9, 18–21, 247
  existence of, 3, 7, 18
  in healthcare workers, 44
  school pressure and, 18–21
  shame and, 41–42
  See also anxiety; depression; stress
mental health support, increasing, 266–67
Michigan, University of, 77
mindfulness, 136, 216–17
MindPeace, 13, 266
mind reading, 130
mindsets, problematic
  as a continuum, 114
  definition of, 97
  development of, xx, 97–98
  emotions and, 121–22
  example of, 95–96
  impostor phenomenon, 110–14, 122
  maladaptive perfectionism, 17, 98–110, 122
  performance as identity, 115–18
  pressure and, xix–xx
  toxic comparison, 119–21, 205, 227
Minnesota Multiphasic Personality Inventory (MMPI), 7
Monitoring the Future survey, 7
Montessori method, 168
motivation, intrinsic, 222–23, 225
Murthy, Vivek, xv, 3, 207

N

Nadel, Eric, 114
National Board of Medical Examiners, 77
National Bureau of Economic Research, 21
National Comorbidity Survey Adolescent Supplement, 50
National Education Association (NEA), 175
National Federation of State High School Associations, 195
National Parent Teacher Association, 175
National Survey of Children's Health, 50
National Survey on Drug Use and Health (NSDUH), xv, 5–6
Nhat Hanh, Thich, 125–26
Nicholson, Mike, 166, 172
Nietzsche, Friedrich, 78
No Child Left Behind (NCLB) Act, 97, 169

O

Obama, Barack, 45
Odgers, Candice, 8
1N5, 13, 266
optimism, 164, 218
overgeneralization, 128
overscheduling, 23–25, 208, 210, 213, 228, 248
oversensitivity, 155

P

The Palpations, 83
parental pressure, xx, 16, 41, 108, 118
parental support
  advocating for your child, 188–89, 214–15
  anxiety and, 60–67
  autonomy and, 229–35
  cognitive restructuring and, 132–41
  college application process and, 186–88
  depression and, 40–41
  extracurricular activities and, 210–15
  goal disruption and, 157–65
  impostor phenomenon and, 112–14
  maladaptive perfectionism and, 108–10
  mitigating school harms through, 181–86
  performance as identity and, 116–18
  self-assessment check of, 185
  toxic comparison and, 119–21
  worry and, 59–60
parent-child relationship, compromised, 208–9
perfectionism
  adaptive, 104, 105–6
  definition of, 98–99
  other-oriented, 99, 108
  self-oriented, 99, 104–6
  socially prescribed, 99
  See also maladaptive perfectionism
performance as identity, 115–18, 134
personalization, 128
Pfau, Liz, 37
planfulness, 163–64
play
  benefits of, 245
  disappearance of free, 3, 4–5, 24, 209–10
  forms of, 245
Pope, Denise, 20
praise, 113–14, 239
PrepMatters, 201–2
pressure
  academic performance and, 87–89
  anxiety and, 50, 68
  burnout and, 206–8, 215–18
  depression and, 9–12
  excessive, xviii–xix, 8–9
  parental, xx, 16, 41, 108, 118
  reducing, 90–91, 248–50
  social media and, 25
  suicide and, 21–23
  teen mental health and, 18–21
  See also stress

R

Race to Nowhere, 13
Ray, Amit, 136
Reggio Emilia approach, 168
relatedness, 222, 228–29, 240–42
resilience curriculum, 79, 84–85
Robert Wood Johnson Foundation, 51
Ryan, Richard, 222

S

Saint Louis University (SLU), xiv–xv, xvii, xxi–xxii, 71–91, 101–2, 115, 122, 132, 136, 221–24, 242, 253–59, 262–63
satisfied nonperfectionism, 104, 106
school curriculum
  acceleration of, 176–77
  narrowing and inflexibility in, 171–72
school refusal, 63
schools
  at-risk kids in, 177–78
  block scheduling and, 178, 180, 263–64
  board, running for, 260–61
  choosing, 189–93
  educational theory and, 167–68
  focused on knowledge acquisition and memorization, 169–70

innovations in, 179–81
later start times for, 264–65
mitigating harms of, at home, 181–86
passive teaching and learning in, 170–71, 179
standardized testing and, 97, 168, 169–70
student autonomy and, 172–73
students' experiences of, 166–69, 179, 219–21
See also academic performance; change; extracurricular activities; grades; homework; school curriculum
self-blame, 128
self-calming, 61–62, 67, 160
self-critical nonperfectionism, 104, 106
self-determination theory, 222–25, 228–29, 242, 245
self-directed learning, 166, 168, 265–66
self-fulfilling prophecy, 129
shame, 41–42
Short Almost Perfect Scale (SAPS), 101
Siegel, Daniel, 207
Siegel, Jason, 150–51, 155
Slaney, Robert, 101
sleep
encouraging, 62, 211
lack of, 16–17, 204–5
later school start times and, 264–65
social media and digital technology, 97, 116
cognitive distortions and, 126
focus on, as source of problems, xviii, 3–5, 8, 262
friendships and, 228
pervasiveness of, 4
pressure and, 25
toxic comparison and, 119, 205, 227
Socrates, xxiii
sports, 195–200, 205, 212–14
"Stanford Ducks," 182–83, 261
Stanford University
applications to, 10–12
Challenge Success, 21
Start Schools Later, 265
State-Trait Anxiety Inventory (STAI), 56
Stixrud, William, 202, 230
Stoicism, 125
stress
burnout and, 206–8, 215–18
causes of, 14–16, 19–21, 53–54, 73–74
external, 53
handling, 77–78
healthy, 55–56
meaning of, 53–54
for parents, 207
reducing, 73–75
research on, 12–21
response, biological, 53, 55–57
toxic, 56
See also pressure
Substance Abuse and Mental Health Services Administration (SAMHSA), 5–6
success log, keeping, 114
suicide
depression and, 39–40
preventing, 39–40
school pressure and, 21–23
Suicide and Crisis Lifeline, vii, 40
timing of, 21–23
surveys, conducting, 262–63
Swierkosz, Jim, 75

T

technology. *See* social media and digital technology
testing, standardized, 97, 168, 169–70
test prep courses, 201–3
therapy
for anxiety, 64–66
for depression, 38–39
thoughts
disputing, 139–41, 145–46, 147–48

thoughts (*cont'd*)
goal expectation violations and, 154–55
labeling, 137–38, 144–45, 147
noticing, 135–37, 144, 146
See also cognitive distortions; cognitive restructuring
Three Good Things practice, 217
travel, 244
tunnel vision, 128–29, 156
tutoring, 201–3
Twenge, Jean, 3, 6–7, 50

U

UCLA, xxii, 33, 78, 215
uncertainty, tolerance for, 164–65
Utah State University, 198

V

Vescelius, Andrea, 181, 242
Village High School, 180
Virginia, University of, 77

W

Wahlstrom, Kyla, 264
Wallace, Jennifer Breheny, 98
water, contaminated, 44–45
withdrawal, 34
World Health Organization, 206
worry, 54, 59–60. *See also* anxiety; catastrophizing

Y

Yerkes, Robert M., 88
Yerkes-Dodson law, 88–89

About the Author

STUART SLAVIN is a board-certified pediatrician and award-winning medical educator and researcher who served most recently as Vice President for Well-Being at the Accreditation Council for Graduate Medical Education (ACGME). Dr. Slavin obtained his MD from Saint Louis University (SLU), then completed his residency training at the University of California, Los Angeles, where he remained as a faculty member for seventeen years. While at UCLA, he earned a master's degree in education (MEd) from the University of Southern California. Dr. Slavin returned to SLU as Associate Dean for Curriculum in 2004, and while there, he led groundbreaking efforts to improve the mental health of medical students, which produced dramatic decreases in rates of depression and anxiety in students while improving academic performance. Over the past decade, Dr. Slavin has been actively engaged in research related to adolescent mental health. He lives in Santa Fe, New Mexico, with his partner and their dog, Little.